The Massachusetts General Hospital Protocols and Procedures for Venous Disease

Carlos Echevarria
Julianne Stoughton
Anahita Dua
Editors

The Massachusetts General Hospital Protocols and Procedures for Venous Disease

Springer

Editors
Carlos Echevarria
Division of Vascular and Endovascular Surgery
Department of Surgery
Massachusetts General Hospital/
Harvard Venous & Lymphatic Medicine Alumni
Boston, MA, USA

Julianne Stoughton
Division of Vascular and Endovascular Surgery
Department of Surgery
Massachusetts General Hospital/
Harvard Medical School
Boston, MA, USA

Anahita Dua
Division of Vascular and Endovascular Surgery
Department of Surgery
Massachusetts General Hospital/
Harvard Medical School
Boston, MA, USA

ISBN 978-3-032-05707-5 ISBN 978-3-032-05708-2 (eBook)
https://doi.org/10.1007/978-3-032-05708-2

This Springer imprint is published by the registered company Springer Nature Switzerland AG
The registered company address is: Gewerbestrasse 11, 6330 Cham, Switzerland

Preface

In the dimly lit scriptorium of the medieval monastery, the air hung heavy with the musty scent of old parchment and the soft murmurs of monks engrossed in their diligent work. The flickering light of a single candle cast eerie shadows on the worn wooden desks and ancient manuscripts that lined the shelves.

Brother Ambrose, a diligent and scholarly monk, hunched over his desk meticulously transcribing a faded text. The silence of the room was shattered when a blood-curdling scream echoed through the cloisters. Monks dropped their quills and rushed toward the source; their faces etched with horror.

As they reached the scene, they discovered Brother Augustine lying lifeless on the cold stone floor, surrounded by a pool of crimson. Gasps of shock filled the air, and the abbot, a stern and authoritative figure, hurried to the gruesome sight.

The initial assumption was murder, as the monastery had been plagued by tensions and disagreements over religious matters. The abbot called for an investigation, and Brother Francesco de Medici, a keen and logical monk renowned for his deductive skills, took charge.

Rumors and whispers spread like wildfire through the monastery as the news of Brother Augustine's untimely death reached every corner. Superstitious beliefs intertwined with the shock and grief, leading some monks to speculate that malevolent spirits or the wrath of God had claimed Brother Augustine's life. The ancient stone walls seemed to echo with fearful murmurs, and anxious glances were exchanged among the brethren, each contemplating the ominous significance of the event.

Brother Francesco, though experienced in unraveling mysteries through reason, found himself navigating the delicate balance between logic and the fervent beliefs that permeated the monastery.

There were no signs of struggle, no weapon, just a trail of blood leading to the lifeless corpse. His eyes were wide open, staring at nothing. His pale face bore an expression of eternal repose, the lines of scholarly contemplation etched into features now frozen in death. The once-vibrant brown robe, stained with the deep hue of his own lifeblood, clung eerily to his motionless frame. A thin trail of crimson seeped from beneath his habit, marking the path of the fatal varicose vein that had unleashed the silent tragedy.

Brother Francesco, despite solving the mystery, couldn't help but ponder the dark irony of a monk's death by a bleeding varicose vein. The Abbey, already haunted by secrets and forbidden knowledge, now bore witness to the silent tragedy of a monk succumbing to an ailment hidden beneath his holy robes.

This book hopes to bring light to the most relevant, and the somewhat obscure, topics of venous and lymphatic disease. This book is written for those who want to learn the art of medicine in venous disease, those who would like to expand their knowledge, and those who would like to standardize their practice with the training, techniques, and protocols used at the Massachusetts General Hospital.

Phoenix, AZ, USA Carlos Echevarria, MD, MMM, FSVM, RPVI

Contents

Part VI Procedures

Contributors

Syed T. Ahsan Division of Vascular Medicine Henry Ford Hospital, Detroit, MI, USA

Ryan T. Brooks Division of Vascular and Endovascular Surgery, Department of Surgery, Massachusetts General Hospital/Harvard Medical School, Boston, MA, USA

Cheryl L. Brunelle Department of Physical and Occupational Therapy, Massachusetts General Hospital, Boston, MA, USA

Syed Moez Shah Bukhari Department of Cardiovascular Disease, Johns Hopkins University, Baltimore, MD, USA

Rui Dai Division of Interventional Radiology, Department of Radiology, Massachusetts General Hospital, Boston, MA, USA

Dania Daye Division of Interventional Radiology, Department of Radiology, Massachusetts General Hospital, Boston, MA, USA

Anahita Dua Division of Vascular and Endovascular Surgery, Department of Surgery, Massachusetts General Hospital/Harvard Medical School, Boston, MA, USA

Carlos Echevarria Division of Vascular and Endovascular Surgery, Department of Surgery, Massachusetts General Hospital/Harvard Venous & Lymphatic Medicine Alumni, Boston, MA, USA

Division of Vascular Medicine and Endovenous Interventions, Veins & Vascular Centers of Excellence, Phoenix, AZ, USA

Jeremy Goverman Department of Surgery, Massachusetts General Hospital, Sumner Redstone Burn Center, Harvard Medical School, Boston, MA, USA

Lynn Gray-Meltzer Department of Physical and Occupational Therapy, Massachusetts General Hospital, Boston, MA, USA

M. Ihsan Kaadan Division of Cardiology, Department of Medicine, Rush University Medical Center, Chicago, IL, USA

Maureen Walsh McCarthy Department of Surgery, Massachusetts General Hospital, Lead NP Wound Service, Boston, MA, USA

Jahan Mohebali Division of Vascular and Endovascular Surgery, Department of Surgery, Massachusetts General Hospital, Boston, MA, USA

Gaurav Parmar Vascular Medicine, Massachusetts General Hospital/Harvard Medical School, Boston, MA, USA

Animan Randhawa Division of Interventional Radiology, Department of Radiology, Massachusetts General Hospital, Boston, MA, USA

Sara Rose-Sauld Department of Foot and Ankle Orthopedics, Massachusetts General Hospital/Harvard Medical School, Boston, MA, USA

Gloria Salazar Department of Radiology, University of North Carolina at Chapel Hill, Chapel Hill, NC, USA

Sherry D. Scovell Division of Vascular and Endovascular Surgery, Department of Surgery, Massachusetts General Hospital/Harvard Medical School, Boston, MA, USA

Reza Seyedsadjadi Department of Neurology – Neuromuscular Medicine, Massachusetts General Hospital/Harvard Medical School, Boston, MA, USA

Julianne Stoughton Division of Vascular and Endovascular Surgery, Department of Surgery, Massachusetts General Hospital/Harvard Medical School, Boston, MA, USA

Luis Suarez Division of Vascular and Endovascular Surgery, Department of Surgery, Massachusetts General Hospital/Harvard Medical School, Boston, MA, USA

Davis Waller Division of Vascular and Endovascular Surgery, Department of Surgery, Massachusetts General Hospital, Boston, MA, USA

Jonathan Winograd Plastic and Reconstructive Surgery, Massachusetts General Hospital Lymphedema Center of Excellence, Boston, MA, USA

Part I

Chronic Venous Insufficiency

Superficial Venous Insufficiency

1

Carlos Echevarria
and Julianne Stoughton

Case/Teaser

Brother Ambrose, the subject of this book introduction, unquestionably had venous insufficiency. The disease carries an increased risk of thrombosis and chronic leg ulcers, and has been associated with poor quality of life and even death. Nonetheless, insufficiency of the superficial venous system remains an obscure topic, little discussed in medical education and poorly understood by the public at large.

The venous network outside the lower limbs' muscular fascia constitutes the superficial venous system. It is represented by a large network of interconnected tributary and truncal veins,

C. Echevarria (✉)
Division of Vascular and Endovascular Surgery, Department of Surgery, Massachusetts General Hospital/Harvard Venous & Lymphatic Medicine Alumni, Boston, MA, USA

Division of Vascular Medicine and Endovenous Interventions, Veins & Vascular Centers of Excellence, Phoenix, AZ, USA
e-mail: carlos.echevarria@vascular.md

J. Stoughton
Division of Vascular and Endovascular Surgery, Department of Surgery, Massachusetts General Hospital/Harvard Medical School, Boston, MA, USA
e-mail: jstoughton@mgh.harvard.edu

C. Echevarria et al. (eds.), *The Massachusetts General Hospital Protocols and Procedures for Venous Disease*,
https://doi.org/10.1007/978-3-032-05708-2_1

largely represented by two large truncal veins: the Great Saphenous Vein (GSV) and the Small Saphenous Vein (SSV). As the surrounding tissue lacks a supportive muscular structure, these veins depend on their multiple valves to help maintain the unidirectional flow of blood toward the heart. Prolonged backflow in any of these veins is described as superficial venous insufficiency.

We use the Clinical-Etiology-Anatomy-Pathophysiology (CEAP) classification to better understand the disease's condition. CEAP is a classification, not a score; higher numbers do not necessarily indicate severity or its impact on patients. However, it categorizes the condition in the clinical context of the disease.

The Clinical Picture

Clinical classification	
C_0	No visible or palpable signs of venous disease
C_1	Telangiectasias or reticular veins
C_2	Varicose veins
C_{2r}	Recurrent varicose veins
C_3	Edema
C_4	Skin and subcutaneous tissue changes secondary to chronic venous disease
C_{4a}	Pigmentation or eczema
C_{4b}	Lipodermatosclerosis or atrophie blanche
C_{4c}	Corona phlebectatica
C_5	Healed ulcer
C_6	Active venous ulcer
C_{6r}	Recurrent active venous ulcer
S	Symptoms attributable to venous disease
A	Absence of symptoms

Although some cases may be clinically silent, a population study found that over 20% of people have some degree of symptomatic venous disease, and the severity of the disease increases with age [1]. The most common symptoms are summarized in the acronym HASTI (Heaviness, Aching, Swelling, Throbbing, Itching). Advanced disease has more prevalent signs, such as notable reticular veins with skin quality changes such as hyperpigmentation or lipodermatosclerosis. This could lead to bleeding varicosities, ulcers, and poor wound healing. The C classification encompasses all these signs and symptoms, yet none are pathognomonic of superficial venous insufficiency. It is the corollary of signs and symptoms as a whole that makes the disease condition. CEAP is meant to be used for venous disease only. Leg swelling may be the expression of venous disease, but patients with other etiologies for edema, including stand-alone lymphedema or lipedema, should *not* be categorized using the CEAP classification. Additionally, patients may present different CEAP classes between legs and within the same limb. As a result, a patient with a swollen limb and hyperpigmentation of the skin should not be labeled as C4a (using the incorrect logic of reporting the highest score) but as C3,4a instead.

HASTI	
H	Heaviness
A	Aching
S	Swelling
T	Throbbing
I	Itching

Etiology of the Disease

Etiologic classification	
Ec	Congenital
Ep	Primary
Es	Secondary
En	No etiology identified

Unlike vascular malformations, venous insufficiency is not typically a congenital condition noted soon after birth. Instead, it has been proposed that certain risk factors predispose to the development of primary venous insufficiency over time. The San Diego population study showed that the most significant risk factors for superficial venous insufficiency are:

Age (OR 1.4–1.6)
Personal or family history of vein disease (OR 2.3–2.9)
Static foot disorders (flat feet OR 1.4–3.4)
Laborers (presumably working long hours in the standing or sitting position OR 1.1–3.2)
Tobacco smoking (OR 2.2) [1]

Anatomy of the Disease

Anatomical classification	
As	Superficial
Ap	Perforator veins
Ad	Deep veins
An	No anatomical location identified

An ultrasound probe placed on the non-weight-bearing extremity with the patient in the standing position is the best study to evaluate for superficial venous insufficiency. The supine position is incorrect for detecting reflux and should only be used to evaluate the deep venous system. However, finding reflux is not enough. Ultrasound findings must correlate with the clinical features to be considered relevant. For example, GSV pathology is usually associated with HASTI symptoms and poor wound healing on the medial surface of the lower leg. SSV pathology may be associated with HASTI, but its treatment does not usually improve *medial* surface wounds. In contrast, venous ulcers on the *lateral* aspect of the calf may benefit from SSV intervention [2]. For pathological perforators, the most recent guidelines have put more emphasis on the skin changes that precede a wound to prevent the development of a non-healing ulcer.

Perforator veins are communicating veins between the superficial and deep venous system. Reversal of flow may still be considered normal. Established guidelines from the American Venous Forum (AVF) and the Society for Vascular Surgery (SVS) define the term "pathologic perforator vein" when there is more than

500 ms of reflux and the diameter of the vein at the fascia level is greater than 3.5 mm. These findings must include surrounding skin changes and active or healed ulceration.

Pathophysiology

Pathophysiological classification	
Pr	Reflux
Po	Obstruction
Pn	No pathophysiology identified

The most crucial pathophysiological feature of venous insufficiency is venous hypertension. Reverse venous return will pool blood by gravity to the lower limbs, increasing pressure in the superficial venous system and engorging truncal veins and their most distal and superficial branches.

When discussing with patients, one can share the analogy of the plumbing system in a house. The heart is the water pump, blood vessels function as the pipelines, and the lungs as the filter within the system. Anything affecting the flow within this circuit could increase pressures and cause venous reflux.

The Pumps

Axial pump function is provided mainly by the heart, but around 90% of the venous return coming from the lower extremities is, in fact, through the action of the plantar and calf muscle venous pumps [3]. As a result, failure of these pumps could cause venous insufficiency independently of cardiac function. When the calf muscles contract, the pressure in the posterior compartment increases significantly, reaching up to 250 mmHg. This ejection function (along with venous valves preventing backward flow) decreases resting venous pressures. Consequently, pressure in the posterior tibial vein drops from 80–100 mmHg to less than 30 mmHg with every pump [4].

The Pipelines

Any obstruction within the venous lumen or extrinsic compression of the vein may elevate venous pressures. It is essential to assess the venous system for signs of thrombosis or restrictive flow. Additionally, conditions outside of venous disease such as congestive heart failure or pulmonary hypertension, may also lead to increased back pressures and lower limb superficial venous insufficiency [5].

Finally, incompetent venous valves may also be a cause of venous hypertension. Bicuspid valves throughout the venous system improve return by interrupting the column of hydrostatic pressure. Failure to do so would inevitably elevate the pressure within the system. This could be due to congenital causes or scarring after venous pathology. Vein enlargement may also increase the distance between valves, causing failure to close. Studies have shown that a GSV diameter of ≥5.1–5.8 mm and an SSV diameter of ≥3.6–5.3 mm have the best positive predictive value for venous reflux [6, 7].

Differential Diagnosis

One must consider alternative etiologies for patients with leg pain, varicose veins, or swollen limbs; most importantly when signs, symptoms, and imaging findings are out of proportion to the degree of pain or swelling. Consider the pattern of disease and alleviating and aggravating factors such as time of day, position, and changes with physical activity. Even in the presence of venous insufficiency, the behavior of the signs or symptoms can be foretelling. For example, patients may have postpartum limb swelling and varicosities after pregnancy. Postpartum limb swelling should resolve within a few weeks after delivery. Should the swelling last more than 3 months, one must consider alternative etiologies [8]. Worsening pain with physical activity must rule out arterial disease or musculoskeletal etiologies. The presence of numbness or tingling might suggest neurologic etiologies.

Conditions such as polyneuropathies, restless leg syndrome, peripheral artery disease, lymphedema, and lipedema could pose a clinical challenge for diagnosis, as they may be concurrently present in patients with superficial venous insufficiency (see Chap. 8).

Diagnosing venous insufficiency requires clinical and imaging findings before planning treatment or intervention. All leg signs and symptoms in addition to all pertinent review of systems must be identified to lead to an accurate diagnosis.

Diagnostic and Management

Auxilliary Testing/Imaging Studies

A functional venous duplex ultrasound must demonstrate reversed venous flow (reflux) with provocative maneuvers. This is done by exerting pressure distal to the probe and monitoring the directionality of the flow during and after the release (see Chap. 12). If this cannot be done, the Valsalva maneuver may show the direction of flow at the deep venous junctions by increasing venous pressure below the diaphragm. The presence of reflux (venous flow coming back toward the probe), greater than 500 ms for superficial or perforator veins or greater than 1000 ms for deep veins, supports the diagnosis of venous insufficiency [9] (Fig. 1.1).

When scanning via duplex ultrasound, it is important to identify changes in the venous flow pattern at and above the saphenofemoral junction (SFJ). Asymmetric venous wave changes, lack of phasicity (respiratory pattern), or pulsatility may constitute indirect findings of more proximal pathology, which may warrant further studies.

We reserve the use of a CT venogram when the venous ultrasound shows the above patterns or when there is high clinical suspicion of disease in the suprainguinal veins. The asymmetric disease burden in the lower limbs, pelvic signs or symptoms, multiple thrombotic episodes, or recurrent treatment failure may warrant further studies. In general terms, we reserve the use of MR

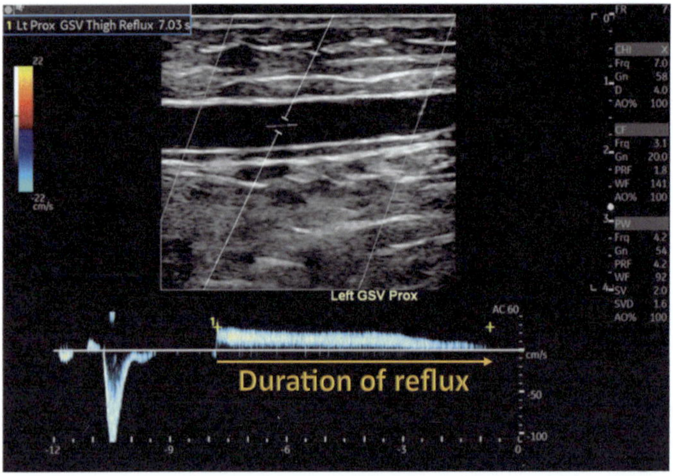

Fig. 1.1 Compression below the probe will generate a first monophasic Doppler waveform (flow going away from the probe). If reflux is present, a second wave opposite to the fist will be recorded (flow coming toward the probe)

venograms for younger patients who can stay still for prolonged periods. In our experience, both modalities are robust diagnostic methods with similar accuracy.

Although venography has been largely replaced by venous ultrasound, its concept is worth mentioning. Descending venography requires proximal injection of contrast with the patient on a tilt table in the vertical position while doing Valsalva. This technique may identify reflux in the common femoral and saphenofemoral junction. Ascending venography visualizes the distal injection of contrast traveling cephalad within the deep venous system in search of pathology.

Management

- ATLANTIS trial (2020): Aquatic therapy vs. control in venous insufficiency
- ESCHAR Study (2004): Effect of surgery and compression on ulcer healing and recurrence
- EVRA Study (2018): Early Venous Reflux Ablation in venous ulceration

Medical Management

In general terms, conservative therapy such as weight loss and exercise, is always recommended. That said, studies on calf ejection fraction have shown deleterious effects of exercise in patients with venous insufficiency who have a limited calf pump function [10]. Leg elevation is of some benefit, provided there is no pinching of the venous system by the groin area that could worsen venous return. Compression stockings with a minimal pressure of 20–30 mmHg offer temporary improvement of symptoms to some people and, in our experience, may render some predictive benefit with future interventions. However, some patients report significant discomfort with their use (frequently in those with associated neuropathic symptoms), limiting their benefit. For such patients, the ATLANTIS trial demonstrated that aquatherapy (15 minutes of walking or swimming in a pool three times a week for three months) might represent an exciting alternative to compression hoses, improving the clinical status and quality of life in patients with chronic venous insufficiency [11]. This is probably due to the compression exerted by water pressure when the limbs are submerged. The elements of conservative therapy should be reviewed and tailored to each patient's specific needs.

The Case for Venoactive Drugs (VADs)

In a 2005 Cochrane Review, the efficacy of all VADs was analyzed and reported in 4413 patients included in 44 published studies and found data to be insufficient to support their use [12]. However, in 2020, the Cochrane group re-examined the data registered prior to this date in 56 studies and 7690 patients. They found that VADs slightly reduce lower extremity edema (RR 0.70, 95%), ankle circumference (mean difference −4.27 mm, 95%) but did very little difference in quality of life (SMD −0.06, 95%) [13]. Karathanos et al. evaluated the role of flavonoids after endovenous thermal ablation and found the benefit equivalent to 1-point reduction in the 1–10 Visual Analog Scale (VAS) for pain [14].

Endovascular/Surgical Interventions

Although treatment of telangiectasias and reticular veins (C1) (<3 mm) is often considered cosmetic in nature, this could lead to an error of judgment as they represent the first signs of superficial venous insufficiency. It is imperative to assess the impact of symptoms on patients' quality of life to determine if treatment is warranted. Clinical indication for treatment becomes evidently appropriate when superficial varicosities represent a significant risk of hemorrhage with minimal trauma, or when their proximity to an active or healed ulcer contributes to local venous hypertension. For patients with C4–C6 disease, including those with varicose bleeding or recurrent superficial thrombophlebitis, conservative management is not sufficient and may require intervention. This was demonstrated first with the ESCHAR study. Subjects underwent saphenofemoral junction disconnection and saphenous stripping. Although ulcer healing rates were not found to be statistically significant, ulcer recurrence rates/ulcer-free time at 4 years were significantly lower in the compression plus surgery group compared with the compression group alone (31% vs. 56%; $P < 0.001$) [15]. With the advent of endovenous techniques, this concept was revisited in the EVRA Study (Early Venous Reflux Ablation in venous ulceration) with ulcers <6 months old. The authors demonstrated faster median ulcer healing times of 56 days (95% CI, 49–66) in the early intervention group vs. 82 days (95% CI, 69–92) in the deferred intervention group [16].

Thermal Ablation

Endovenous Laser Ablation Therapy (EVLT)

EVLT is done by introducing a laser fiber via percutaneous Seldinger technique (needle over a wire) to ablate incompetent superficial veins.

Multiple semiconductor (diode) laser wavelengths have been tested, including 810, 940, 980, 1064, 1320, and 1470 nm. Although some studies have shown less postoperative pain with the 1470 nm fibers, data has been conflicting, and the success rate is similar regardless of the wavelength used [17, 18].

The axial veins are the primary target for this therapy (GSV, SSV, and ASV). The fiber tip must be identified 2 cm from the junction and, with the patient in the Trendelenburg position, the laser fiber is steadily pulled to deliver approximately 40 J/cm.

Pathological perforator veins are the most common cause of recurrent venous insufficiency. Their treatment is indicated when the following criteria are met:

1. Surrounding skin changes harbinger of venous ulcers, or venous ulcers per se
2. No saphenous reflux (or previously treated)
3. Reverse flow of >500 ms from deep to superficial venous system
4. Minimal diameter of 3.5 mm (measured along the fascia)

It is usually recommended to treat axial veins first, as addressing GSV insufficiency may resolve perforator reflux. A case for treatment of perforator veins with C2 disease can be made when no GSV pathology preceded these findings, or there is a recurrence of disease despite GSV treatment (although some health insurances may challenge it). Perforator veins can be challenging when placing a guidewire, as there is limited purchase of vein length to hold the wire in place. Instead, an 18G IV catheter needle may be used under ultrasound guidance. A bare laser fiber perfectly fits into the 18G sheath snuggled into the vein (Fig. 1.2).

Radiofrequency Ablation (RFA)

RFA is a minimally invasive percutaneous technique similar to EVLT. However, rather than having a direct heating element, the friction of the oscillating molecules affected by radiofrequency energy emits heat, affecting the cells of the incompetent vein interior walls.

The indications for treatment are the same as for other ablation techniques. The catheter should be placed 2 cm below the junction. Verify this with ultrasound after tumescent anesthesia, as the catheter may move forward after perivenous fluid allocation. The RF catheter tip can be up to 10 cm in length. Therefore, treatments are done by segments rather than continuous pulling, as done with laser fibers. Unlike lasers, RF requires segment compression during ablation by either the ultrasound probe or manual compression.

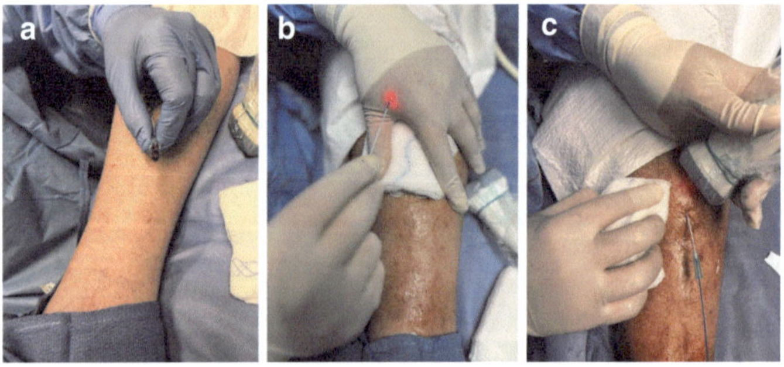

Fig. 1.2 Once the 18G IV sheath is in the perforator vein (**a**), the laser fiber replaces the access needle (**b**). Advancing the fiber beyond the point of resistance at the sheath tip assures laser function without damaging the sheath in place. Proper laser fiber placement is always confirmed by ultrasound before treatment (**c**). (Courtesy: Carlos Echevarria, MD)

Severe tortuosity of a vein segment may pose a challenge for thermal techniques, as the passage of the device may not be feasible. Manual external compression and knee bending may improve the passage. If this fails, multiple access points may overcome this challenge. Also, skillful placement of tumescent anesthesia may improve the advancement of the device. The injection of tumescent can also create a buffer layer of protection from thermal injury to the surrounding tissue when the vein in question comes out of fascia and lies superficial <1 cm from the skin surface.

A national registry study demonstrated the average tumescent anesthesia volume used for thermal methods is approximately 5 cc/cm of treated vein. We found a correlation between lower volumes of tumescent anesthesia and increased risk of recanalization, especially when the volume used is less than 135 cc. We believe this to be associated with the limited reduction of vein diameter when low volumes of tumescent anesthesia are used during treatment [19].

Non-Thermal Ablation

Sclerotherapy

Sclerotherapy is the eighteenth-century technique of injecting chemical irritants into pathological veins. Although there are over 20 different sclerosant agents, they can all be classified into four distinct categories: thrombogenics, detergents, osmotics, and chemical irritants per se. Regardless of their classification, they share a common objective: endothelial damage of the venous wall. However, agent selection, concentration, and state (liquid vs. foam) will impact the balance between effectiveness and complications. Because of the extravasation of the agent beyond the vein wall, the most common side effects are skin irritation and ulcer formation. Some patients may also have post-sclerotherapy skin hyperpigmentation due to hemosiderin accumulation. Most of these complications self-resolve over time, but in some cases it could take up to 1–2 years.

- Liquid Sclerosant:
  Liquid sclerotherapy is the treatment of choice for telangiectasias, reticular veins, and small varicose veins. In the United States, it is convention and common practice to use Polidocanol 0.5% for veins 1–3 mm and 1% for veins 3–5 mm. We usually reserve sodium tetradecyl sulfate at 3% for more prominent varicosities, especially in the pelvis (ovarian and periuterine veins). Upon contact with blood, most sclerosants are deactivated within 2 seconds. However, this may be enough time to develop thrombosis, especially in those with a prior history. In those cases, we recommend a brief period of prophylactic anticoagulation.
- Foam Sclerosant: Ultrasound-Guided Foam Sclerotherapy (UGFS):
  In 2001, Tessari et al. developed a technique where 1 part of a sclerosant agent and four parts of room air were mixed multiple times through a 3-way stopcock [20]. The physician-compunded foam displaces blood in larger veins (rather than mixing with it) while increasing the contact surface area and time exposure of the sclerosant to the venous endothelium (Fig. 1.3). The technique requires immediate injection to avoid foam breakdown. To overcome this, a patented formula of low-

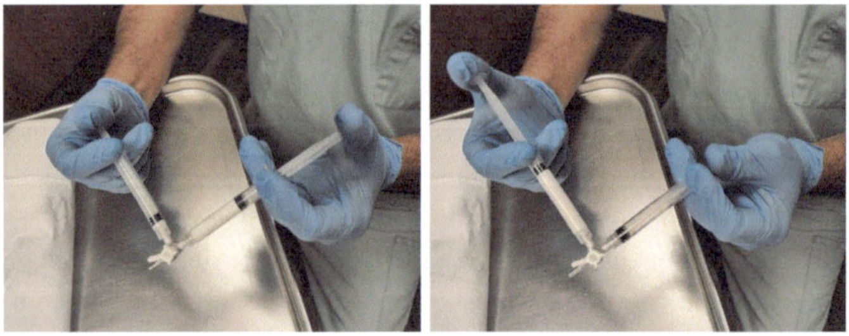

Fig. 1.3 Tessari technique requires 10–20 mixing attempts to produce a thick foam. Note in the picture that the stopcock valve may be turned slightly off/misaligned to decrease the aperture and create a thicker foam. (Courtesy: Carlos Echevarria, MD)

nitrogen (<0.8%), O2:CO2 (65:35 ratio) foam was created. Polidocanol 1% endovenous microfoam (Varithena®) is almost twice the time more stable than physician-compounded foams [21]. Foam preparations are commonly indicated for treating symptomatic varicose veins ≥3 mm in diameter.

Chemical Adhesive (Cyanoacrylate Embolization)

Cyanocrylate, a fast-acting adhesive with multiple medical and non-medical uses, was first patented by B.F. Goodrich in 1947. However, there was a pause on its medical use due to its potential to cause skin irritation. Now, newer formulations are believed to be more innocuous and are currently used for occlusion of incompetent veins and venous malformations. This method is an excellent alternative for those patients who express concerns about tolerating pain. Unlike thermal ablation, this non-thermal method does not require multiple needle injections for tumescent anesthesia and causes no postoperatory pain. It induces a foreign body reaction for venous closure, so there are risks of hypersensitivity reaction and granuloma formation at the puncture exit site [22, 23]. A retrospective study found that C3 and C4 classification, younger age, and active smoking status contribute significantly to the risk of type IV hypersensitivity reaction [24]. In our practice, we avoid it altogether if the patient has a history of allergies or in episfascial saphenous veins with a depth of <1 cm as the fibrosis caused may become palpable in such cases.

Mechanochemical Ablation (MOCA)

This technique uses the simultaneous effect of mechanical injury of a rotating wire and the chemical injury of a liquid sclerosant. This method does not require tumescent anesthesia or causes post-operatory pain. Although uncommon, we have seen patients feeling pain when the wire gets stuck in the venous internal wall, as in a valve, or when the vein is close to the skin.

Surgical: Ligation, Stripping, Phlebectomy

With the advent of thermal and non-thermal techniques, saphenous vein stripping and high ligation have fallen out of favor due to their risk of neovascularization. Histopathology studies have demonstrated that after 6 weeks of dissecting the GSV, highly irregular new venous vessels reconnect the previously transected ends of the saphenous vein. After 40 weeks there is complete reconstitution of venous flow [25].

Microphlebectomy, also known as stab phlebectomy, removes superficial varicosities through a small 1–2 mm skin incision overlying the vein. We like to perform the incision with a beveled-point 18-gauge filter needle rather than a scalpel, avoiding a more extensive laceration or a more profound wound. Then, we fish the vein through the hole with small curved hemostatic forceps or vein hooks, keeping a steady pull traction until most of the varicose vein has been removed. Note that if this method is done after using a sclerosant agent, veins may become friable and more challenging to remove in one piece (Table 1.1).

Table 1.1 Recommendations and special considerations for different superficial venous ablation methods

	Recommended	Special considerations
Thermal methods (EVLT/RF)	Truncal vein >12 mm	Caution with treatment of GSV below the knee (risk of saphenous nerve damage)
MOCA	Truncal vein <8–10 mm	Avoid in recanalized veins or a history of thrombosis
Cyanocrylate glue	Aversion to needles	Glue may be palpable in epifascial axial veins or tributaries. Use polydocanol endovenous microfoam (PEM) in glue recanalization
PEM	Tortuous incompetent axial veins	Treated epifascial veins may cause skin hyperpigmentation and phlebitis of tributaries
Ambulatory microphlebectomy	Epifascial tributaries	May leave small scar. Avoid in certain areas such as lateral knee (risk of peroneal nerve damage)

Surveillance

We usually follow up within 3 days after sclerotherapy/Polidocanol 1% endovenous microfoam (Varithena®) or 7 days after all other ablation techniques. We use the revised VCSS to assess treatment outcomes [26]. Our goal is to assess symptoms, offer proper dressing changes and wound care, and rule out potential complications. We recognize that the incidence of post-ablation thrombotic events is 1.3–1.7% [27], so we consider performing a follow-up ultrasound on those with risk factors or symptoms of concern. This appointment may miss potential type IV hypersensitivity reactions from cyanoacrylate as they usually appear around 2 weeks after exposure. These events may be captured during telephone encounters or at the first-month visit.

Complications and Management

The most concerning complication aside from post-procedural pain is hyperpigmentation and thrombosis. Although we dedicate two chapters to venous thrombosis, post-procedural thrombosis warrants special consideration.

Ablation Related Thrombus Extension (ARTE, Formally EHIT) [28]

It is paramount that the tip of the device used, whether thermal or non-thermal, is identified and followed with ultrasound. This must be verified multiple times, if needed, before initiating treatment. It is not unheard of that when advancing a guidewire, this could inadvertently enter a perforator and lie in the femoral vein instead. Identifying the junction, fascia, and surrounding anatomy is the best way to avoid complications of this nature. Thrombosis of the femoral vein above the junction could happen due to microtrauma from the guidewire or catheter advancement. Thrombus may not be contiguous to the treated vein and may require anticoagulation (Table 1.2).

Table 1.2 Ablation-related thrombus extension (ARTE) is a complication of endovenous ablation therapies

	Definition	Treatment	Surveillance
Class I	Thrombus without propagation up to deep vein junction	None	None
Class II	Thrombus propagation <50% deep vein lumen	None	Weekly
Class III	Thrombus propagation >50% deep vein lumen	Anticoagulation until resolution	Weekly
Class IV	Occlusive DVT extending from the treated vein	Anticoagulation for a minimum of 3 months as per DVT guidelines	

Ablation-related thrombus extension (ARTE) is a revised term that includes endothermal heat-induced thrombosis (EHIT) and other types of thrombus extension due to chemical and mechanical techniques. Regardless of etiology, the management is defined by its degree of propagation

Class I asymptomatic Isolated distal deep vein thrombosis in the soleal or gastrocnemius veins after venous treatment is unlikely to propagate, but may be considered judicious to follow up with weekly ultrasounds. Anticoagulation is initiated if the thrombosis becomes highly symptomatic or is indicated by any of the following: evidence of Acute Thromboembolism (ARTE) class changes, extensive thrombus propagation, ablation-related thrombus extension (e.g., >5 cm or involving multiple veins), concerning risk factors, or a positive D-dimer.

Key Point Synopsis

I feel this chapter could be best summarized by reviewing the case of Brother Ambrose. Without additional information about his condition, we can safely state he had at least a C2 classification, and assuming no prior history of thrombosis, he would be C2EpAsPr (this is a superficial venous insufficiency chapter after all). We can infer that Brother Ambrose's risk factors may have been his long sedentary hours of transcribing old texts and possibly his loose monk sandals (poorly fit footwear can alter gait parameters and potentially affect venous pump flow).

As many Spanish monasteries were burned during the Spanish Civil War in the 1900s, it is fair to say that Brother Ambrose episode happened anytime before these dates. Compression stockings were not invented until 1950; therefore, his options for conservative management would be naturally occurring flavonoids like horse chestnut, and aquatherapy. Should the bleeding had been noted on time, our recommendation would have been to elevate his leg and apply finger-point pressure to the varicosity until the bleeding stopped.

Since sclerosant agents were first developed in the eighteenth century, he could have benefited from direct treatment of the bleeding varicosity, which to this day remains the standard of care for these cases. Nowadays, once the acute event is controlled, patients benefit from modern medicine with proper diagnostic ultrasounds and ablation therapy of the source truncal vein.

Summary

Insufficiency of the superficial venous system remains an obscure topic, little discussed in medical education and poorly understood by the public at large. This chapter organizes the topic based on the Clinical-Etiology-Anatomy-Pathophysiology (CEAP) classification to understand the disease's condition and discuss differential diagnosis. Other conditions, such as limb swelling and neuropathy, pose a clinical challenge for diagnosis, as they may be concurrently present, leaving superficial venous insufficiency underdiagnosed and undertreated for years. Studies have demonstrated that early venous reflux ablation not only prevents late-stage venous ulcer disease but also promotes healing when present. This chapter discusses different ablation methods, indications, and contraindications.

References

1. Criqui MH, Denenberg JO, Bergan J, Langer RD, Fronek A. Risk factors for chronic venous disease: the San Diego Population Study. J Vasc Surg. 2007;46(2):331–7. https://doi.org/10.1016/j.jvs.2007.03.052. Epub 2007 Jun 27. PMID: 17600666; PMCID: PMC2023874.
2. Bass A, Chayen D, Weinmann EE, Ziss M. Lateral venous ulcer and short saphenous vein insufficiency. J Vasc Surg. 1997;25(4):654–7. https://doi.org/10.1016/s0741-5214(97)70291-x.
3. Pollack AA, Wood EH. Venous pressure in the saphenous vein at the ankle in man during exercise and changes in posture. J Appl Physiol. 1949;1:649.
4. Ludbrook J. The musculovenous pumps of the human lower limb. Am Heart J. 1966;71:635–41.
5. Aldemir M, Emren SV, Balçık Ç, Onrat E, Gürsoy M. Primary pulmonary arterial hypertension with preserved right ventricular function leads to lower extremity venous insufficiency. Vascular. 2018;26(2):183–8. https://doi.org/10.1177/1708538117723201. Epub 2017 Aug 23. PMID: 28835185.
6. Joh JH, Park HC. The cutoff value of saphenous vein diameter to predict reflux. J Korean Surg Soc. 2013;85(4):169–74. https://doi.org/10.4174/jkss.2013.85.4.169. Epub 2013 Sept 30. PMID: 24106683; PMCID: PMC3791359.
7. Choi JY, Lee J-H, Kwon OJ. Association between the saphenous vein diameter and venous reflux on computed tomography venography in patients with varicose veins. PLoS One. 2022;17(2):e0263513. https://doi.org/10.1371/journal.pone.0263513.
8. Berks D, Steegers EAP, Molas M, Visser W. Resolution of hypertension and proteinuria after preeclampsia. Obstet Gynecol. 2009;114(6):1307–14. https://doi.org/10.1097/AOG.0b013e3181c14e3e. PMID: 19935034.
9. Labropoulos N, Tiongson J, Pryor L, et al. Definition of venous reflux in lower-extremity veins. J Vasc Surg. 2003;38:793–8.
10. Mosti G, Partsch H. Improvement of venous pumping function by double progressive compression stockings: higher pressure over the calf is more important than a graduated pressure profile. Eur J Vasc Endovasc Surg. 2014;47(5):545–9, ISSN 1078-5884. https://doi.org/10.1016/j.ejvs.2014.01.006.
11. Sharifi M, Bay RC, Karandish K, Emrani F, Snyder R, D'Silva S, ATLANTIS Trial. The randomized, controlled ATLANTIS trial of aquatic therapy for chronic venous insufficiency. J Vasc Surg Venous Lymphat Disord. 2021;9(4):961–70. https://doi.org/10.1016/j.jvsv.2020.10.016. Epub 2020 Oct 28. PMID: 33127467.
12. Martinez-Zapata MJ, Bonfill Cosp X, Moreno RM, Vargas E, Capellà D. Phlebotonics for venous insufficiency. Cochrane Database Syst Rev. 2005;(3):CD003229. https://doi.org/10.1002/14651858.CD003229.

13. Martinez-Zapata MJ, Vernooij RW, Simancas-Racines D, Uriona Tuma SM, Stein AT, Moreno Carriles RMM, Vargas E, Bonfill Cosp X. Phlebotonics for venous insufficiency. Cochrane Database Syst Rev. 2020;11(11):CD003229. https://doi.org/10.1002/14651858.CD003229.pub4. PMID: 33141449; PMCID: PMC8094625.
14. Karathanos C, et al. Prospective comparative study evaluating the role of flavonoids after endovenous thermal ablation. Phlebology. 2021;36(8):644–50.
15. Barwell JR, Davies CE, Deacon J, Harvey K, Minor J, Sassano A, Taylor M, Usher J, Wakely C, Earnshaw JJ, Heather BP, Mitchell DC, Whyman MR, Poskitt KR. Comparison of surgery and compression with compression alone in chronic venous ulceration (ESCHAR study): randomised controlled trial. Lancet. 2004;363(9424):1854–9. https://doi.org/10.1016/S0140-6736(04)16353-8. PMID: 15183623.
16. Gohel MS, Heatley F, Liu X, Bradbury A, Bulbulia R, Cullum N, Epstein DM, Nyamekye I, Poskitt KR, Renton S, Warwick J, Davies AH, EVRA Trial Investigators. A randomized trial of early endovenous ablation in venous ulceration. N Engl J Med. 2018;378(22):2105–14. https://doi.org/10.1056/NEJMoa1801214. Epub 2018 Apr 24. PMID: 29688123.
17. Doganci S, Demirkilic U. Comparison of 980 nm laser and bare-tip fibre with 1470 nm laser and radial fibre in the treatment of great saphenous vein varicosities: a prospective randomised clinical trial. Eur J Vasc Endovasc Surg. 2010;40(2):254–9. ISSN 1078-5884, https://doi.org/10.1016/j.ejvs.2010.04.006, https://www.sciencedirect.com/science/article/pii/S1078588410002625.
18. El-Sheikha J, et al. A prospective observational study comparing early clinical outcomes of 810nm and 1470nm endovenous laser ablation in the treatment of superficial venous insufficiency. Ann Vasc Surg. 2015;29(4):642–3.
19. Echevarria C, Scovell S, Blebea J, Thornton M, Stoughton J. Clinical outcomes following treatment for small saphenous vein insufficiency: an AVLS PRO venous registry study. Phlebology. 2025;40:518–27.
20. Tessari L, Cavezzi A, Frullini A. Preliminary experience with a new sclerosing foam in the treatment of varicose veins. Dermatologic Surg. 2001;27(1):58–60.
21. Carugo D, Ankrett DN, Zhao X, Zhang X, Hill M, O'Byrne V, Hoad J, Arif M, Wright DD, Lewis AL. Benefits of polidocanol endovenous microfoam (Varithena®) compared with physician-compounded foams. Phlebology. 2016;31(4):283–95. https://doi.org/10.1177/0268355515589063. Epub 2015 Jun 1. PMID: 26036246; PMCID: PMC4838175.
22. Yie K, Shin AR, Jung EH, Hwang EJ. Incidence and clinical impact of endovenous glue-induced hypersensitivity among patients who underwent endovenous cyanoacrylate ablation procedures: a registry-based cohort study. Dermatologic Surg. 2023;49(8):783–9. https://doi.

org/10.1097/DSS.0000000000003849. Epub 2023 May 29. PMID: 37249557.

23. Sumarli SA, Lee QWS, Yap HY, Tay HTL, Chong TT, Tang TY. Exit site complications following cyanoacrylate glue endovenous ablation of incompetent truncal veins for chronic venous insufficiency. J Vasc Surg Cases Innov Tech. 2020;6(4):500–4. https://doi.org/10.1016/j.jvscit.2020.08.010. PMID: 33134630; PMCID: PMC7588813.
24. O'Banion LAA, Shao MY, Ali A, Kochubey M, Yan Y, Fallentine J, Oh JH, Patel HR, Agrawal N, Carmona E, Hager ES, Kiguchi MM. Type IV hypersensitivity reaction after cyanoacrylate venous closure. Ann Vasc Surg. 2023;95:218–23. ISSN 0890-5096, https://doi.org/10.1016/j.avsg.2023.06.002, https://www.sciencedirect.com/science/article/pii/S0890509623003151.
25. Glass GM. Neovascularization in restoration of continuity of the rat femoral vein following surgical interruption. Phlebology. 1987;2(1):1–6. https://doi.org/10.1177/026835558700200106.
26. Gloviczki P, Comerota AJ, Dalsing MC, et al. The care of patients with varicose veins and associated chronic venous diseases: clinical practice guidelines of the Society for Vascular Surgery and the American Venous Forum. J Vasc Surg. 2011;53(5):2S–48S.
27. Gloviczki P, et al. The 2023 Society for Vascular Surgery, American Venous Forum, and American Vein and Lymphatic Society clinical practice guidelines for the management of varicose veins of the lower extremities. Part II. J Vasc Surg Venous Lymphat Disord. 2024;12(1):101670.
28. Kabnick LS, et al. Classification and treatment of endothermal heat-induced thrombosis: recommendations from the American Venous Forum and the Society for Vascular Surgery. J Vasc Surg Venous Lymphat Disord. 2021;9(1):6–22. https://doi.org/10.1016/j.jvsv.2020.06.008.

Deep Venous Insufficiency

2

Rui Dai, Animan Randhawa, Dania Daye,
Davis Waller, and Jahan Mohebali

Case/Teaser

A 48-year-old man presents to the Interventional Radiology clinic with symptomatic left calf varicosities, leg fatigue, and swelling for 2 years. His symptoms are exacerbated by ambulation, standing for long periods at work as a dentist, and playing tennis. He has been using prescription-strength compression stockings for several years with minimal relief. He does not have any significant past medical or surgical history. He does not smoke cigarettes or use any illicit drugs. He has no family history of venous insufficiency/varicose veins, venous/arterial malformations, coagulopathy, or thrombophilia. On physical exam, he has multiple 3–4 mm varicosities in the medial left calf and a painful, large 6 mm varicosity in the posterior left thigh.

R. Dai · A. Randhawa · D. Daye (✉)
Division of Interventional Radiology, Department of Radiology, Massachusetts General Hospital, Boston, MA, USA
e-mail: rdai@mgh.harvard.edu; arandhawa2@mgh.harvard.edu; ddaye@mgh.harvard.edu

D. Waller · J. Mohebali
Division of Vascular and Endovascular Surgery, Department of Surgery, Massachusetts General Hospital, Boston, MA, USA
e-mail: Mohebali.Jahan@mgh.harvard.edu

C. Echevarria et al. (eds.), *The Massachusetts General Hospital Protocols and Procedures for Venous Disease*,
https://doi.org/10.1007/978-3-032-05708-2_2

Anatomy of the Disease

Deep venous insufficiency (DVI) is a chronic disease that develops due to failure of the deep venous system, leading to venous hypertension and valvular reflux. Deep venous insufficiency may be broadly classified into primary and secondary subtypes. The pathophysiology of each subtype is discussed in detail below.

- *Primary venous insufficiency* is due to inherent defects in valves or venous walls, frequently associated with congenital defects such as valvular agenesis or connective tissue disorders. There is no precipitating event in primary venous insufficiency. Abnormalities in the venous walls include reduced elastin content, inflammatory infiltration, and increased extracellular matrix remodeling. These factors compromise the integrity of the veins and promote dilation and incompetence of the venous valves. This is typically seen in conditions such as Klippel-Trenaunay syndrome, Parkes-Weber syndrome, and other congenital venous malformations.
- *Secondary venous insufficiency* is preceded by a causative event due to the subsequent damage to venous valves or walls. Precipitating events include thrombosis, proximal venous obstruction (which may be non-thrombotic), lifestyle factors, medications, trauma, and hormonal changes. Prior thrombotic events can trigger a cellular and humoral response in the affected vein, which can lead to vascular remodeling, causing the vein to become chronically occluded or severely stenotic. This, combined with associated signs and symptoms such as leg heaviness, swelling, and chronic wounds, represents a condition known as post-thrombotic syndrome (PTS).

It is essential to review the anatomy of the venous system to understand the development and progression of deep venous insufficiency.

The veins of the lower extremity may be divided into superficial, deep, and perforating veins. The superficial veins can be subdivided into collecting veins characterized by thin walls or truncal veins that are thick-walled, such as the Great Saphenous Vein (GSV). The GSV drains into the deep venous system via the saphenofemoral junction (SFJ). The deep veins of the lower extremity include the plantar vein, the paired peroneal, anterior, and posterior tibial veins, and the popliteal and femoral veins. The perforating veins communicate with both the superficial and deep venous systems and are important for the equilibration of blood flow.

The veins of the lower extremity must counteract the forces of gravity, hydrostatic pressure, and intra-abdominal pressure to return blood to the heart. Depending on the anatomy of the patient, extrinsic venous compression may represent an additional force, for instance, as in May-Turner syndrome, where the natural path of the right iliac artery may compress the left iliac vein. Venous return to the heart is aided by squeezing the calf muscles, preventing reflux by venous valves, and bidirectional flow of blood via the perforating veins.

Venous valves divide blood into segments of hydrostatic columns, ensure cephalad blood flow, and minimize force on the distal veins. Incompetence of venous valves can, therefore, lead to reflux. Patients with deep venous insufficiency typically will also develop superficial venous insufficiency due to perforating vein valvular failure, which leads to higher pressure in the superficial veins, thereby preventing the complete closure of valves in the superficial system.

Clinical Presentation

Patients with DVI may present with lower extremity edema, leg heaviness and aching, itching, cramping, varicose veins, venous claudication, skin hyperpigmentation, and ulcers. Venous ulcers are the most severe manifestation of chronic DVI and lead to significant morbidity [2].

Risk factors for the development of deep venous insufficiency include female gender, aging, pro-thrombotic conditions such as the use of oral contraceptive pills, pregnancy, smoking, obesity, sedentary lifestyle, trauma, and prior history of deep venous thrombosis [1].

Differential Diagnosis

The differential diagnosis for deep venous insufficiency usually encompasses the differential for lower extremity edema. This includes acute deep venous thrombosis (DVT), congestive heart failure, liver disease, endocrine disorders, renal insufficiency, lymphedema, musculoskeletal injury, compartment syndrome, and side effects of medications. In addition, patients presenting with lower extremity ulcers must be evaluated for other underlying causes or superimposed infections.

May-Thurner Syndrome

Virchow (of Virchow's Triad fame) was one the first physicians to recognize and publish on the association between iliofemoral vein thrombosis and left leg laterality when he stated that thrombotic events were five times more likely to occur in the left leg than the right [31]. Nearly a century later, May and Thurner's published results from their studies on 430 cadavers found that 22% had left iliac vein compression between the right iliac artery and fifth lumbar vertebra (Fig. 2.1) [32]. Today, this is corroborated with high resolution axial imaging. In one recent study, 25% of participants were found to have >50% asymptomatic compression of the left iliac vein [33]. This same study found that the left iliac vein was compressed by the right iliac artery 84% of the time [33]. However, some cases of venous compression may result in inflow venous hypertension, valvular incompetence, or venous insufficiency. Patients with symptomatic iliac vein compression are typically female, in the second to fourth decade of life, and the compression most often manifests with iliofemoral DVT or persistent unilateral lower extremity edema.

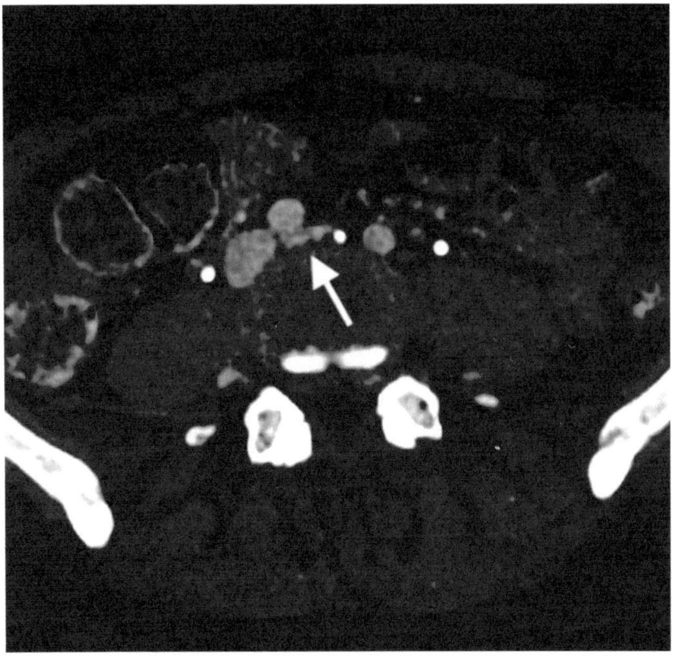

Fig. 2.1 A 17-year-old female with a family history of factor V Leiden mutation presents following excruciating pain after standing up from a seated crossed-leg position and was found to have extensive left lower extremity deep venous thrombosis. CTV demonstrates narrowing of the left iliac vein by greater than 50% (arrow) by the overlying right iliac artery

Diagnosis

Evaluation of deep venous insufficiency warrants a thorough history taking, including the presence, severity, and duration of symptoms. Medical history of comorbidities, medication use, prior episodes of venous thrombosis, surgical history (especially recent interventions), social history including sedentary lifestyle, and family history including coagulopathies. Although we may be tempted to use the Clinical-Etiology-Anatomy-Pathophysiology

(CEAP) classification to quantify the severity of venous disease, CEAP is a categorical classification. The Venous Clinical Severity Score (VCSS) may be better suited to assess the severity of the condition and long-term treatment outcomes [3].

Physical examination includes visual inspection and palpation of the affected extremity. Ideally, the patient should be standing upright for maximum distension of veins. Historically, maneuvers with a tourniquet while performing a Trendelenburg test were the best initial tests for evaluating superficial and deep venous insufficiency. The patient first empties the venous system by elevating the lower extremity. Then, a tourniquet is applied below the SFJ junction before the patient is positioned upright. In patients with superficial venous reflux, the varicose veins distal to the tourniquet will remain collapsed. In patients with deep venous reflux, varicose veins will immediately reappear upon standing. The Perthes test requires the patient to walk for 5 min or stand up and down on their toes ten times. This maneuver should increase deep venous return and empty the engorged superficial varicosities. Failure to do so would be a sign of deep venous insufficiency [4].

More sophisticated yet noninvasive tools, such as venous Doppler ultrasound, are typically used to assess the great saphenous vein, the small saphenous vein, and their primary tributaries. Ultrasound can identify acute and prior venous thrombosis, the presence of reflux, the duration of reflux, and an anatomic map to delineate levels of involvement, as well as variant anatomy. A reflux time greater than 0.5 s for superficial veins and 1.0 s for deep veins is used to diagnose the presence of reflux [3].

Advanced imaging techniques such as magnetic resonance venogram (MRV) or computed tomography venogram (CTV) can also be used to evaluate the etiology of deep venous insufficiency further. For instance, it can be used to identify complex variant anatomy such as May-Thurner. While there is no significant difference in MRV and CTV for proximal venous imaging to delineate anatomical compression or collateralization, MRV does offer some benefits, namely, reduced radiation exposure flow-sensitive sequencing improve timing for optimal visualization (Fig. 2.2). It can also suggest the hemodynamic significance of venous compression by demonstrating retrograde flow in the ipsilateral iliac

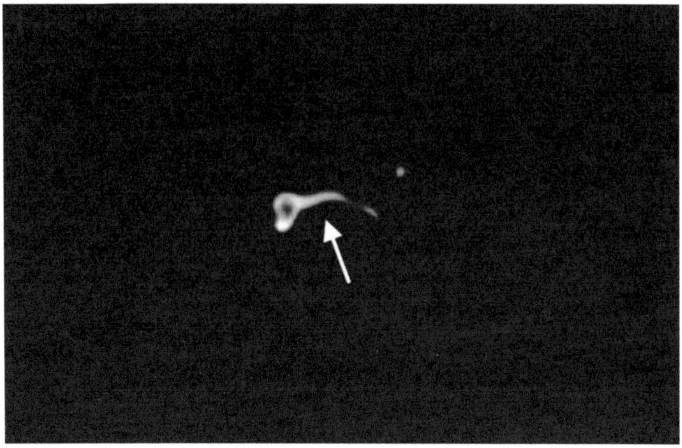

Fig. 2.2 A 44-year-old female with a past medical history of discoid lupus erythematous presents for MR angiogram evaluation of May-Thurner anatomy in the setting of isolated left lower extremity edema. Fluid-sensitive MR sequence clearly demonstrates a moderate narrowing of the left iliac vein

vein [34]. The greatest disadvantage is table time, affecting image quality due to patient motion as frequently seen in those with a history of back pain or the elderly.

Invasive testing, such as contrast venography and intravascular ultrasound, can also be used to evaluate the morphology of the deep venous system and guide treatment.

Medical Management

- CAVENT trial (2012): PTS after CDT in iliofemoral vein thrombosis
- ATTRACT trial (2016): PTS after CDT in iliofemoral vein thrombosis
- CAVA trial (2020): PTS after CDT in iliofemoral vein thrombosis
- VDIO trial (2017): Venogram vs. IVUS in iliofemoral obstruction

For most patients with chronic DVI, conservative treatment with compression stockings and anticoagulation therapy for thrombotic cases is sufficient. Early detection of DVI is essential to the success of conservative treatments. However, for some patients who have disease refractory to medical management or extensive thrombus burden, surgical or interventional thrombolysis, stenting, or valvuloplasty may be required. Prompt initiation of treatment can reduce long-term complications and prevent irreversible changes [5].

For patients with DVI secondary to deep venous thrombosis (DVT), numerous inpatient and outpatient anticoagulation therapies are commonly used depending on the patient's circumstances. Please refer to the DVT chapter for further information.

Endovascular and Surgical Interventions

In patients with DVI secondary to DVT and with contraindications to systemic anticoagulation or extensive thrombus burden, symptomatic conservative management alone may be insufficient. Many surgical and minimally invasive options have been demonstrated to be safe and effective in different clinical circumstances.

Percutaneous Mechanical Thrombectomy

Mechanical thrombectomy can be performed via open surgery or endovascularly with percutaneous mechanical thrombectomy (PMT). Surgical thrombectomy removes the target thrombus through an external excision. Because of the level of invasiveness needed for surgical thrombectomy, there is more significant morbidity compared to endovascular thrombectomy. Surgical thrombectomy is, therefore, often reserved for extensive thromboses that are inaccessible endovascularly.

PMT can be based on aspiration or mechanical fragmentation. Mechanical fragmentation of the thrombus creates a direct passage through the clot via physical clot disruption. Compared to thrombus aspiration, mechanical fragmentation is significantly faster. However, there is a risk of internal vessel injury and further damage to the venous valves, depending on the mechanism of fragmentation. One of the most common mechanisms is rotational thrombectomy, which sheers and macerates the target thrombus with a sinusoidal wire. Several case series in patients with deep venous thrombosis following mechanical thrombectomy with Cleaner XT™ (Argon Medical Devices; Plano, TX, USA) demonstrated approximately 90% technical success and 60% clinical success rates [10, 11].

Other mechanical fragmentation devices manually core and separate the thrombi from the vessel walls, such as ClotTriever BOLD™ (Inari Medical; Irvine, CA, USA). Rheolytic thrombectomy, such as AngioJet (Boston Scientific; Natick, MA, USA) and JETi™ (Abbott; Irvine, CA, USA), injects jets of high-pressured saline to break the thrombi and vacuum the fragments into a catheter. All have been demonstrated to have effective clot reduction; however, the exact rates differ depending on the study and associated patient population [12–14]. Other noncommercialized devices are also available, such as one that combines mechanical fragmentation and aspiration by sequestering the thrombus with a balloon on either side of the target [15].

Aspirational thrombectomy evacuates thrombi by generating a negative intraluminal pressure. However, suction collapses the venous walls, which can dislodge distal thrombi outside the device's negative pressure zone and result in distal pulmonary emboli. Collapse of the vessel walls can also damage the inner vessel lumen, increasing the risk of post-procedural thrombose recurrence. Studies of several existing aspirational thrombectomy devices, such as Indigo (Penumbra, Inc.; Alameda, CA, USA) and AngioVac (AngioDynamics; Latham, NY, USA), found that they have comparable technical and clinical success rates as mechanical thrombectomy [16, 17]. The main differences in benefits between fragmentation and aspirational thrombectomy appear to depend on the size of the thrombus and associated vessels. Because of the large-bore cannula required for aspirational thrombectomy devices, devices such as AngioVac are most effective for thrombi in large vessels. In contrast, fragmentation thrombectomy seems to be better for smaller vessel thrombi.

Catheter-Directed Thrombolysis (CDT)

Systemic thrombolysis with streptokinase, urokinase, or tissue plasminogen activator is generally avoided because of the risk of unintended bleeding and the practicability of local thrombolytic delivery with CDT. This therapy consists of locally infusing thrombolytic agents close to the thrombi for pharmacological disruption of the clot. Prior studies have found that there is no significant difference in overall inpatient mortality between CDT plus systemic anticoagulation versus anticoagulation alone [18]. CDT, however, is associated with significantly higher rates of intracranial hemorrhage compared to anticoagulation alone. Therefore, CDT is absolutely contraindicated in patients with recent neurosurgery, intracranial trauma, or active internal bleeding [19].

Theoretically, it is possible to exclusively use CDT to dissolve thrombi with minimal clot perturbation or vessel injury locally. Still, practically, in most clinical settings, PMT is often performed in combination with CDT to increase technical success, especially if CDT alone initially fails to resolve the clot. A retrospective study that examined CDT with or without PMT found that there is no significant difference in the rate of postoperative complications [20].

Localized directed treatment of DVT decreases the risk of systemic bleeding and decreases the time to thrombolysis. However, it does not reduce the risk of developing post-thrombotic syndrome (PTS). Although the CAVENT trial showed a statistically significant reduction of PTS [6], the ATTRACT and CAVA trials questioned this findings [7, 8]. Perhaps this statement warrants further explanation. Although CAVENT and ATTRACT had a 6% absolute risk reduction of moderate to severe PTS in the CDT+anticoagulation arm compared to anticoagulation only, the bulk of patients developed just mild PTS in both groups. In fact, only 1 of 89 patients with anticoagulation in the CAVENT trial had severe PTS at the 5-year follow-up, and almost half of those used warfarin at subtherapeutic levels. Notwithstanding these findings, additional analysis has yielded important insights:

- Although the incidence of PTS may not be affected, the severity of PTS was significantly reduced in CDT patients.
- These benefits extended to those patients with iliofemoral thrombosis only; those with femoropopliteal DVT did not benefit from CDT.
- CDT patients >65 years old were at greater risk of bleeding and developing PTS compared to younger patients.

Venous Stenting

Endovascular stents can be used to relieve the site of obstruction for targeted areas of proximal venous stenosis, such as in May-Thurner Syndrome. In patients with DVT contributing to DVI, stenting is recommended to restore an acceptable diameter of the venous lumen when PMT, CDT, and venoplasty are insufficient to relieve the stenosis. In patients with extensive iliocaval DVT, iliocaval reconstruction with stenting may be required.

In patients with symptomatic non-thrombotic left common iliac vein lesion (NIVL) leading to DVI, venography with IVUS is undertaken to evaluate the extent of compression. Venous stenting is recommended for patients with a stenosis greater than 61% of the *diameter* (not the area) of the common iliac vein when crossed by the right common iliac artery. This was characterized in the VIDIO trial as follows:

1. When compared to IVUS, venography underestimates stenosis by an average of 11%
2. IVUS was 26% more sensitive than venography in identifying significant lesions (>50%)
3. Treatment of NIVL did not correlate with the area of stenosis. Patients with C4–C6 disease experienced better outcomes from stent treatment when the diameter of stenosis was >61% [9]

Iliac vein stenting for NIVLs has been shown to have superior long-term patency compared to stenting for a thrombotic indication. Many of the publications previously mentioned used the

WallStent as the primary endoprosthesis. Today, there are other, venous-specific stent options and research on outcomes associated with these stents is ongoing. Overall, stenting for NIVL indication is safe with major complication rates <2% [35]. Primary patency at 4 years has been reported up to 98.7% and primary-assisted patency 100% [36]. A NIVL stenting large series review reported that anticoagulation was unnecessary postoperatively and aspirin does not affect patency [37]. However, this particular topic is still a matter of debate. At our institution, patients are prescribed dual antiplatelet therapy for at least 3 months post-stenting and will remain on at least one antiplatelet medication for life, although regimens vary. Higher-risk patients, including those with history of VTE, active malignancy, or diagnosed thrombophilia, will be prescribed an anticoagulant as well.

Surgical Valvuloplasty

In patients with primary DVI or those with damaged valves secondary to DVT, reconstruction of venous valves with internal or external surgical valvuloplasty can be considered [21]. Internal valvuloplasty excises redundant valves and sutures the edge of each valve cusp to the venotomy site to create a single competent valve. External valvuloplasty identifies the valve attachment lines through the vein wall and sutures the valvular attachment sites to decrease the vein diameter and commissural valve angle. External banding of the veins with a Dacron or polytetrafluoroethylene cuff can also decrease venous diameter to further approximate the valves. Several case series have found symptomatic improvement following surgical valvuloplasties [22], but there is limited evidence to fully validate the clinical outcomes [23].

Valvular transplantation or translocation with prosthetic valves has also been described, but they are limited by technical difficulty and the quality of donor or prosthetic valves. Too much laxity, excessive tension, or unintended valvular torsion following transplantation can all contribute to the incompetency of the transplanted valves and subsequent thrombosis. To date, almost all completed clinical trials with bioprosthetic valves have found unacceptably high rates of thrombosis and failure within 12 months [24].

Bypass Surgery

Open surgery for iliac vein compressive lesions is an alternative if there is failure of endovascular treatment. Open interventions require a surgical bypass to reroute venous inflow around the obstruction to restore venous outflow. It is employed for unilateral iliofemoral venous obstruction and requires a patent contralateral iliofemoral segment [38]. Contralateral saphenous vein is dissected free of distal attachments and is re-oriented and tunneled to the ipsilateral involved iliac vein complex where it is anastomosed to a point distal to the iliac vein lesion. This allows venous inflow from the ipsilateral leg to cross to the uninvolved contralateral side bypassing the outflow obstruction. The Palma procedure has shown to have a cumulative patency of 75% at 5 years.

Surveillance and Complications

Following medical and interventional treatment of DVI, patients should be monitored for changes in symptoms and complications related to the procedures such as:

- Stent migration—In the event of stent migration, consider retrieval and re-stenting with larger size
- Stenting across the profunda vein—Consider additional anti-platelet/anticoagulant to ensure additional prophylaxis against in-stent thrombosis
- In-stent thrombosis—Endovenous thrombectomy and potential stent re-lining

One of the most debilitating sequelae associated with CVI is PTS [25]. Even after medical and interventional treatment, residual remaining thrombi can continue to impede blood flow and result in inflammation that permanently damages remaining venous valves. This culminates in valvular incompetence and venous hypertension, which is associated with the pathophysiology of PTS [26].

Several attempts have failed to devise a predictive tool for PTS. Notwithstanding, the Villalta scale [27], Ginsberg measurement [28], the Clinical Etiology Anatomic Pathophysiologic (CEAP) classification, and the Venous Clinical Severity Score (VCSS) further classify patient symptoms following treatment interventions and provide some guidance on disease progression in these patients [29, 30].

In our practice, after intervention of iliac vein compression, we will see the patient in clinic within 4–6 weeks with a venous duplex ultrasound and CTV. These diagnostic tests allow us to assess venous flow both dynamically and statically and determine if there is any acute stent or graft compromise. Additionally, we can assess the patient's symptomatic improvement. Assuming there are no complications, the patient will be seen every 3–6 months until 1 year post-intervention and then annually thereafter. Venous duplex studies are the most common surveillance modality used, and additional axial imaging can be obtained if the duplex suggests stent compromise or the patient reports symptoms of concern.

Teaser Case Follow-Up

The patient we presented at the beginning of this chapter was further evaluated with a duplex venous ultrasound. This showed significant deep venous reflux, as illustrated in Fig. 2.3. In the absence of a prior history of DVT, further workup with an MRV assessing for proximal venous obstruction or stenosis revealed May-Thurner syndrome (Fig. 2.4). Venography with IVUS revealed 72% compression of the left common iliac vein. The patient was treated with left common iliac vein stenting, which led to the resolution of DVI on follow-up ultrasound and marked improvement in the left lower extremity swelling with a decrease in the size of the previously noted varicose veins.

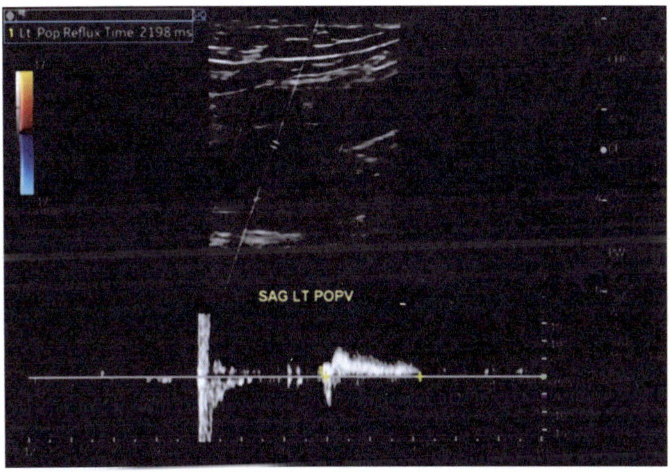

Fig. 2.3 The patient's lower extremity venous duplex ultrasound is notable for significant reflux within the popliteal vein, characterized by a popliteal reflux time of 2.1 s

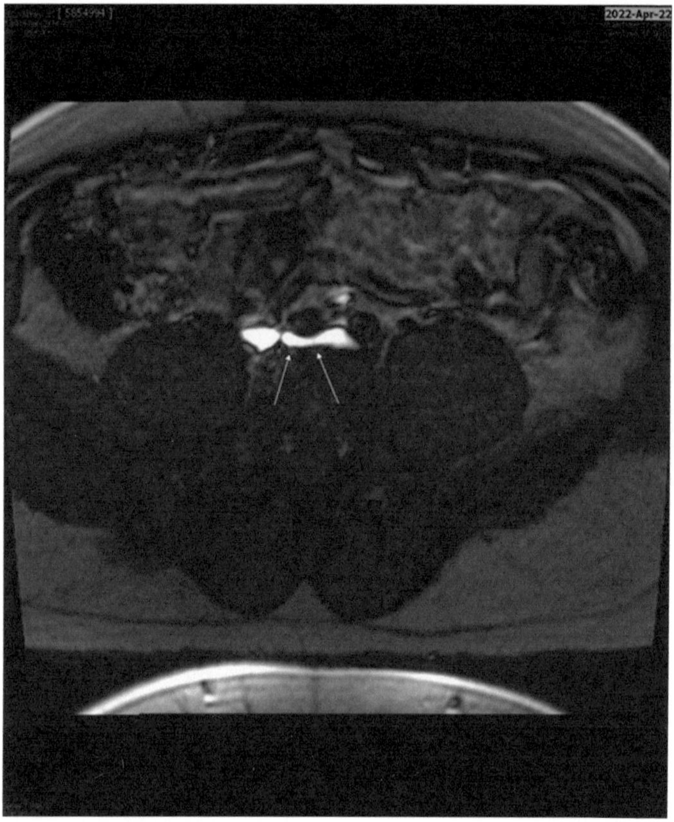

Fig. 2.4 On the MRV for the patient above, there is extrinsic compression of the left common iliac vein by the adjacent crossing of the right common iliac artery, a setting referred to as May-Thurner anatomy. The compression reduces the lumen of the left common iliac vein by over 50%. Not depicted below are collateral veins in the pelvis and a reversed/decreased signal in the left internal iliac vein. This suggests that the compression is hemodynamically significant

Conclusion

DVI is a complex disease that has a wide range of clinical presentations. Treatment also ranges from conservative symptomatic management, pharmacologic anticoagulation, and thrombolysis to surgical valvuloplasty. Here, we present a broad overview of the pathophysiology of chronic DVI and current treatment options.

Summary

Deep venous insufficiency (DVI) is a chronic disease of the lower extremity venous system that can cause debilitating symptoms with serious consequences, including pain, swelling, skin ulcers, nonhealing wounds, and varicose veins. It is a complicated disorder that is often underdiagnosed. There are many causes of DVI, and depending on the etiology of the disorder, different treatment strategies can be employed. Advanced imaging techniques such as computed tomography or magnetic resonance venogram can be used to characterize different complex anatomic variants that can cause DVI. Treatments range from conservative compression stockings and oral anticoagulation to minimally invasive procedures such as percutaneous thrombolysis and stenting. Surgical venous bypass and valvuloplasty are possible in patients with refractory disease. The purpose of this chapter is to provide a general overview of common causes of DVI and different imaging techniques that can be used to determine the underlying etiology, followed by different interventional and surgical treatment options, each with a different set of advantages and disadvantages.

References

1. Maurins U, Hoffmann BH, Lösch C, Jöckel K-H, Rabe E, Pannier F. Distribution and prevalence of reflux in the superficial and deep venous system in the general population—results from the Bonn Vein Study, Germany. J Vasc Surg. 2008;48:680–7.
2. Baliyan V, Tajmir S, Hedgire SS, Ganguli S, Prabhakar AM. Lower extremity venous reflux. Cardiovasc Diagn Ther. 2016;6:533–43.
3. Eberhardt RT, Raffetto JD. Chronic venous insufficiency. Circulation. 2014;130:333–46.
4. Gahtan V, Costanza M. Essentials of vascular surgery for the general surgeon. New York: Springer; 2015.
5. Santler B, Goerge T. Chronic venous insufficiency – a review of pathophysiology, diagnosis, and treatment. J Dtsch Dermatol Ges. 2017;15:538–56.
6. Enden T, Haig Y, Kløw NE, Slagsvold CE, Sandvik L, Ghanima W, Hafsahl G, Holme PA, Holmen LO, Njaastad AM, Sandbæk G, Sandset PM, CaVenT Study Group. Long-term outcome after additional catheter-directed thrombolysis versus standard treatment for acute iliofemoral deep vein thrombosis (the CaVenT study): a randomised controlled trial. Lancet. 2012;379(9810):31–8. https://doi.org/10.1016/S0140-6736(11)61753-4. Epub 2011 Dec 13. PMID: 22172244.
7. Haig Y, Enden T, Grøtta O, Kløw NE, Slagsvold CE, Ghanima W, Sandvik L, Hafsahl G, Holme PA, Holmen LO, Njaaastad AM, Sandbæk G, Sandset PM, CaVenT Study Group. Post-thrombotic syndrome after catheter-directed thrombolysis for deep vein thrombosis (CaVenT): 5-year follow-up results of an open-label, randomised controlled trial. Lancet Haematol. 2016;3(2):e64–71. https://doi.org/10.1016/S2352-3026(15)00248-3. Epub 2016 Jan 6. PMID: 26853645.
8. Notten P, ten Cate-Hoek AJ, Arnoldussen CWKP, et al. Ultrasound-accelerated catheter-directed thrombolysis versus anticoagulation for the prevention of post-thrombotic syndrome (CAVA): a single-blind, multicentre, randomised trial. Lancet Haematol. 2020;7:e40–9.
9. Gagne PJ, Tahara RW, Fastabend CP, Dzieciuchowicz L, Marston W, Vedantham S, Ting W, Iafrati MD. Venography versus intravascular ultrasound for diagnosing and treating iliofemoral vein obstruction. J Vasc Surg Venous Lymphat Disord. 2017;5(5):678–87. https://doi.org/10.1016/j.jvsv.2017.04.007. Epub 2017 Jun 28. PMID: 28818221.
10. Benarroch-Gampel J, Pujari A, Aizpuru M, Rajani RR, Jordan WD, Crawford R. Technical success and short-term outcomes after treatment of lower extremity deep vein thrombosis with the ClotTriever system: a preliminary experience. J Vasc Surg Venous Lymphat Disord. 2020;8:174–81.

11. Moriarty JM, Rueda V, Liao M, Kim GHJ, Rochon PJ, Zayed MA, et al. Endovascular removal of thrombus and right heart masses using the AngioVac system: results of 234 patients from the prospective, multicenter Registry of AngioVac Procedures in Detail (RAPID). J Vasc Interv Radiol. 2021;32:549–557.e3.
12. Ismail U, Rowe RA, Cashin J, Genin GM, Zayed MA. Multimodal thrombectomy device for treatment of acute deep venous thrombosis. Sci Rep. Nature Publishing Group. 2022;12:5295.
13. Lopez R, DeMartino R, Fleming M, Bjarnason H, Neisen M. Aspiration thrombectomy for acute iliofemoral or central deep venous thrombosis. J Vasc Surg Venous Lymphat Disord. 2019;7:162–8.
14. Robertson B, Neville E, Muck A, Broering M, Kulwicki A, Kuhn B, et al. Technical success and short-term results from mechanical thrombectomy for lower extremity iliofemoral deep vein thrombosis using a computer aided mechanical aspiration thrombectomy device. J Vasc Surg Venous Lymphat Disord. 2022;10:594–601.
15. Brailovsky Y, Yeung H-M, Lakhter V, Zack CJ, Zhao H, Bashir R. In-hospital outcomes of catheter-directed thrombolysis versus anticoagulation in cancer patients with proximal deep venous thrombosis. J Vasc Surg Venous Lymphat Disord. 2020;8:538–544.e3.
16. López-Núñez JJ, Trujillo-Santos J, Monreal M. Management of venous thromboembolism in patients with cancer. J Thromb Haemost. 2018;16:2391–6.
17. Loss L, Stefanopoulos S, Siddiq A, Markowiak S, Qu W, Osman M, et al. Catheter directed lysis and thrombectomy are equally effective for extensive deep vein thrombosis. J Surg Res. 2019;244:540–6.
18. D'Addario J, Smeds MR, Wittgen C. Surgical treatment of deep venous insufficiency and requirements for novel interventions. JVS-Vasc Insights. 2023;1:100011.
19. Verma H, Srinivas R, George RK, Tripathi RK. Reduction internal valvuloplasty is a new technical improvement on plication internal valvuloplasty for primary deep vein valvular incompetence. J Vasc Surg Venous Lymphat Disord. 2014;2:383–9.
20. Goel RR, Hardy SC, Brown T. Surgery for deep venous insufficiency. Cochrane Database Syst Rev. John Wiley & Sons, Ltd. 2021;(9):CD001097. Available from: https://www.cochranelibrary.com/cdsr/doi/10.1002/14651858.CD001097.pub4/full.
21. Pavcnik D, Uchida B, Kaufman J, Hinds M, Keller FS, Rösch J. Percutaneous management of chronic deep venous reflux: review of experimental work and early clinical experience with bioprosthetic valve. Vasc Med. SAGE Publications Ltd STM. 2008;13:75–84.
22. Vedantham S. Thrombectomy and thrombolysis for the prevention and treatment of postthrombotic syndrome. Hematology Am Soc Hematol Educ Program. 2017;2017:681–5.

23. Berk BC, Abe JI, Min W, Surapisitchat J, Yan C. Endothelial atheroprotective and anti-inflammatory mechanisms. Ann N Y Acad Sci. 2001;947:93–109; discussion 109–111.
24. Kahn SR. Measurement properties of the Villalta scale to define and classify the severity of the post-thrombotic syndrome. J Thromb Haemost. 2009;7:884–8.
25. Ginsberg JS, Hirsh J, Julian J, Vander LaandeVries M, Magier D, MacKinnon B, et al. Prevention and treatment of postphlebitic syndrome: results of a 3-part study. Arch Intern Med. 2001;161:2105–9.
26. Eklöf B, Rutherford RB, Bergan JJ, Carpentier PH, Gloviczki P, Kistner RL, et al. Revision of the CEAP classification for chronic venous disorders: consensus statement. J Vasc Surg. 2004;40:1248–52.
27. Vasquez MA, Rabe E, McLafferty RB, Shortell CK, Marston WA, Gillespie D, et al. Revision of the venous clinical severity score: venous outcomes consensus statement: special communication of the American Venous Forum Ad Hoc Outcomes Working Group. J Vasc Surg. 2010;52:1387–96.
28. Arko FR, Davis CM III, Murphy EH, Smith ST, Timaran CH, Modrall JG, et al. Aggressive percutaneous mechanical thrombectomy of deep venous thrombosis: early clinical results. Arch Surg. 2007;142:513–9.
29. Wang W, Sun R, Chen Y, Liu C. Meta-analysis and systematic review of percutaneous mechanical thrombectomy for lower extremity deep vein thrombosis. J Vasc Surg Venous Lymphat Disord. 2018;6:788–800.
30. Tang T, Chen L, Chen J, Mei T, Lu Y. Pharmacomechanical thrombectomy versus catheter-directed thrombolysis for iliofemoral deep vein thrombosis: a meta-analysis of clinical trials. Clin Appl Thromb Hemost. 2019;25:1076029618821190.
31. Virchow R. Uber die Erweiterung Kleinerer Gefasse. Arch Path Anat. 1851;3:4279. https://doi.org/10.1007/BF01960918.
32. May R, Thurner J. The cause of the predominantly sinistral occurrence of thrombosis of the pelvic veins. Angiology. 1957;8(5):419–27.
33. Kibbe MR, Ujiki M, Goodwin AL, Eskandari M, Yao J, Matsumura J. Iliac vein compression in an asymptomatic patient population. J Vasc Surg. 2004;39(5):937–43.
34. Butros SR, Liu R, Oliveira GR, Ganguli S, Kalva S. Venous compression syndromes: clinical features, imaging findings and management. Br J Radiol. 2013;86(1030):20130284. https://doi.org/10.1259/bjr.20130284.
35. Seager MJ, Busuttil A, Dharmarajah B, Davies AH. Editor's choice—A systematic review of endovenous stenting in chronic venous disease secondary to iliac vein obstruction. Eur J Vasc Endovasc Surg. 2016;51(1):100–20.
36. Ye K, Lu X, Li W, Huang Y, Huang X, Lu M, Jiang M. Long-term outcomes of stent placement for symptomatic nonthrombotic iliac vein compression lesions in chronic venous disease. J Vasc Interv Radiol. 2012;23(4):497–502.

37. Raju S. Best management options for chronic iliac vein stenosis and occlusion. J Vasc Surg. 2013;57(4):1163–9.
38. Dua A, Heller J, Lee C. Management of post-traumatic phlegmasia cerulea dolens via right-to-left femoral vein to femoral vein bypass (Palma procedure). Vasc Endovasc Surg. 2017;51(8):567–71.

Part II

Thrombosis

Superficial Vein Thrombosis 3

Sherry D. Scovell

Case Summary

The patient is a 55-year-old female with a past medical history significant for superficial venous insufficiency and varicose veins. One week ago, she noticed pain in the varicose veins on the medial aspect of the calf. Over the course of the next several days, she developed increased pain with new redness overlying these veins. The veins, which were compressible, became hard and non-compressible.

Superficial Vein Thrombosis (SVT)

Anatomy of Disease

Superficial vein thrombosis is defined as thrombus and inflammation in the axial superficial venous system. In the lower limbs, these axial superficial veins include the great saphenous vein, the

S. D. Scovell (✉)
Division of Vascular and Endovascular Surgery, Department of Surgery, Massachusetts General Hospital/Harvard Medical School, Boston, MA, USA
e-mail: sscovell@mgh.harvard.edu

C. Echevarria et al. (eds.), *The Massachusetts General Hospital Protocols and Procedures for Venous Disease*,
https://doi.org/10.1007/978-3-032-05708-2_3

small saphenous vein, and the anterior accessory saphenous vein. Thrombus and inflammation may also be present in tributary varicose veins associated with one of the axial superficial veins. If the thrombus is confined to the tributary veins and *not* present in the axial superficial veins, it is referred to as phlebitis or thrombophlebitis. The distinction between the two entities is important, as SVT of the saphenous veins has the strongest association with venous thromboembolism [1, 2].

In a large community-based study from France, the incidence of superficial vein thrombosis has been quoted as 0.64 per 1000 person-years [3]. Although initially believed to be a more common clinical entity, this incidence is approximately half that of DVT and closer to the incidence of pulmonary embolism (PE) [4].

Differential Diagnosis

Superficial vein thrombosis is often confused with lower extremity cellulitis because of the diffuse erythema and tenderness. When superficial vein thrombosis is present in the superficial veins of the calf, it is easier to distinguish as the erythema is overlying a vein. However, when the superficial vein thrombosis is in the thigh, there is more subcutaneous tissue between the vein and the skin, making it more difficult to distinguish it from cellulitis and determine the proximal extent of the inflammation. SVT shares some of the same symptoms as DVT, such as unilateral lower extremity edema and pain, which should be on the differential diagnosis. Lymphangitis, ruptured medial head of the gastrocnemius muscle, tendonitis, popliteal fossa cyst, and hematoma may present with symptoms similar to SVT.

Diagnostic and Management

Auxiliary Testing/Imaging Studies

Following physical examination, venous duplex ultrasound is the initial diagnostic test of choice. The venous duplex ultrasound should always include an evaluation of the entire deep venous system of the lower limb for evidence of DVT. There are three large observational studies evaluating the risk of concurrent venous thromboembolism at the time of diagnosis of SVT: the POST trial documented a 23.5% risk of DVT [5], the OPTIMEV trial a 28.8% risk of DVT [6], and the STEPH trial a 24.6% risk of DVT [3]. It is important to note that the POST and STEPH trials further stated that 40% of these concurrent DVT were proximal DVT and not contiguous with the SVT [7].

At the time of the diagnosis, the rate of symptomatic pulmonary embolism (PE) in these trials ranged from 3.9% to 6.8% [7]. In another trial by Verlato and colleagues, the rate of asymptomatic PE may be as high as 33% [8], underscoring the importance of inquiring about symptoms associated with PE, such as shortness of breath or chest pain.

A lower extremity venous duplex ultrasound for thrombosis and patency should be performed on all patients who present with SVT [9]. This study includes transverse grayscale images without and with transducer compressions (when anatomically possible). These images must be documented and include images of the following veins at a minimum: common femoral vein (CFV), saphenofemoral junction (SFJ), proximal femoral vein, mid femoral vein, distal femoral vein, popliteal vein, peroneal veins, and posterior tibial veins. The anterior tibial vein thrombosis is an extremely uncommon finding [10]. When thrombosis of the anterior tibial vein is noted, it is typically in conjunction with popliteal, posterior tibial, or peroneal vein thrombosis. Therefore, the anterior tibial vein is not typically imaged as part of a lower extremity venous duplex ultrasound for thrombosis and patency. When clinically relevant, additional images are warranted to document areas of suspected thrombosis, such as in the gastrocnemius, soleal, and superficial veins. Additionally, symptomatic axial superficial veins, such as the great saphenous vein, small saphenous vein, anterior accessory saphenous vein, and varicosities in areas of pain and tenderness, should be imaged and documented. When identified, superficial vein thrombosis must be reported, including the name of the involved veins, tributary involvement, if noted, thrombus distance from the junction of the deep venous system at the saphenofemoral or saphenopopliteal junction, and additional images, such as the length of the thrombus. These details are essential in determining treatment options and for documentation should the patient complain of potential propagation. If the thrombus is located near an incompetent perforating vein, patency of that perforating vein should also be documented.

As perforating veins connect the deep and superficial venous systems, it is critical to ensure that there is no thrombus propagation from the superficial into the deep venous system. This typically happens when the perforating veins are incompetent. However, any incompetent perforating veins in proximity to the superficial vein thrombosis should be imaged.

Spectral Doppler waveforms to demonstrate spontaneous venous flow, phasicity, and flow augmentation, where anatomically appropriate, must be documented in the following vessels at a minimum: right and left common femoral veins and the popliteal vein. Abnormalities require additional images and waveforms [9].

D-dimer seems to be unreliable in the diagnosis of SVT. In one study, the sensitivity of D-dimer for the diagnosis of SVT was 74.3%, with a specificity of 43.3% and a positive predictive value of 15.7% [11]. Another prospective database from a DVT service noted that 16% of patients with SVT had an elevated age-adjusted D-dimer, but 6% of patients with SVT had a normal age-adjusted D-dimer [12]. Overall, it may be useful to follow D-dimer over time, but it does not seem helpful in diagnosing this condition.

Management

CALISTO trial (2010)	Placebo vs. Prophylactic dose fondaparinux 45 days. Low risk patients.
SUPRPISE trial (2017)	Prophylactic dose rivaroxaban vs. Prophylactic dose fondaparinux 45 days. High risk patients.
INSIGHTS-SVT trial (2023)	Late thromboembolism risk factors after SVT

Prophylactic anticoagulation should be initiated for acute isolated SVT greater than 5 cm in length and greater than 3 cm from the junction of the deep veins.

The data from the CALISTO trial, which is a large volume, prospective, randomized trial in a low-risk population of patients, demonstrates that prophylactic dose fondaparinux (compared to placebo) administered for 45 days offers an 85% risk reduction of the composite outcome of symptomatic PE, symptomatic DVT, symptomatic SVT recurrence, and symptomatic SVT extension (3 cm or less from the SFJ) [13].

The SURPRISE trial was a phase 3b, non-inferiority prospective, randomized trial that compared prophylactic dose rivaroxaban with prophylactic dose fondaparinux for 45 days in a high-risk population [14]. All patients enrolled had symptomatic isolated SVT plus one risk factor, with 50% having either a history of venous thromboembolism or SVT. Rivaroxaban was found to be non-inferior to fondaparinux for the treatment of acute, isolated SVT. However, the overall composite outcome of symptomatic PE, DVT, SVT recurrence, and thrombus extension was much higher at day 90 compared with the follow-up at day 77 in the CALISTO trial, suggesting that in a patient population at high risk for thrombosis, a longer course of treatment is likely required to decrease future risk of thrombosis.

More recently, the INSIGHTS-SVT, a prospective observational trial, confirmed that the risk of future venous thromboembolism remains high for at least 3–12 months following the acute SVT [15]. It also noted certain risk factors in patients with late events, such as obesity, a history of prior thrombosis, or concurrent infections. These data suggest that in patients with SVT and thrombotic risk factors, extending the duration of prophylactic dose anticoagulation beyond 45 days is warranted to decrease future thrombotic events.

Data on low molecular weight heparin (LMWH—i.e., enoxaparin, dalteparin) shows that subsequent thrombotic events are higher with LMWH than fondaparinux and rivaroxaban [15]. Additionally, from earlier trials, LMWH reduced the extension and recurrence rate of SVT but did not decrease the rate of future DVT or PE [16]. Based on these trials, LMWH is not a first line treatment for SVT, with the exception of pregnancy. LMWH is the preferred anticoagulant in pregnancy based on current evidence-based guidelines, as LMWH does not cross the placenta. The prophylactic dosing of enoxaparin is 40 mg SQ daily. There are no other randomized controlled trials using other direct oral anticoagulants in the treating of SVT.

The prophylactic dosing for SVT is as follows:

- Fondaparinux 2.5 mg SQ daily for 45 days
- Rivaroxaban 10 mg PO daily for 45 days

In addition to prophylactic-dose anticoagulation, superficial vein thrombosis in a patient without superficial venous insufficiency or varicose veins deserves special attention. A search for an underlying etiology for the thrombosis is warranted, including a hypercoagulable workup and screening for occult malignancy. Patients should be up to date on their routine cancer screenings, such as mammography, gynecological examination, and colonoscopy for women and colonoscopy and prostate screening for men,. Additional testing should be undertaken as warranted for occult malignancy based on individual patient risk factors.

If the thrombus is within 3 cm of the deep veins (between the superficial vein and the deep vein or within a perforating vein), patients should be treated with therapeutic dose anticoagulation for 3 months, similar to treatment of DVT [17]. If the thrombus is within the axial superficial veins, less than 5 cm long, and greater than 3 cm from the junction, serial duplex ultrasound should be performed to document propagation under close clinical follow-up. This is especially important when the thrombus is located within the thigh portion of the great saphenous vein, as the propagation of the thrombus may not be accompanied by overlying erythema or pain due to the increasing depth between the skin and the vein as it moves cephalad.

If the thrombus is situated in tributary varicose veins and not within the axial superficial vein and less than 5 cm in length, conservative management with NSAIDs, warm or cool compresses (depending upon the acuity of the thrombus), leg elevation, and compression stockings. Patients should be educated to watch for the propagation of thrombus, which typically translates as pain or redness moving proximally. If patients experience signs or symptoms of propagation, a follow-up duplex ultrasound is warranted to delineate the extent and location of the thrombus and consideration is given to prophylactic dose anticoagulation.

Surgical Management

As the majority of patients have superficial vein insufficiency as the underlying etiology for their SVT, a venous reflux ultrasound to evaluate the superficial venous system for evidence of reflux is appropriate following the acute thrombotic period. In the absence of superficial venous insufficiency and varicose veins, SVT represents a more concerning etiology, such as occult malignancy or thrombophilia. This venous ultrasound is typically performed three months after the acute SVT to allow the acute inflammatory period to resolve and the vein to recanalize.

Recurrence of superficial vein thrombosis occurs in approximately 10% to 20% of patients [17, 18]. To prevent recurrent episodes of SVT, definitive treatment of the axial superficial venous incompetence is appropriate. Endovenous methods of superficial vein closure may be undertaken, such as thermal ablation, with radiofrequency or laser, or non-thermal ablation, with cyanoacrylate adhesive. If there is significant webbing or synechiae within the lumen of the affected vein, chemical ablation with polidocanol endovenous microfoam is a more advantageous option, as passing a catheter or laser fiber proximally may pose a challenge. Mechanochemical ablation should be avoided as the rotating wire on the catheter may become entangled in the regions of webbing and present a challenge to dislodge. Debulking of associated large tributary varicose veins either simultaneously or in a staged manner is appropriate to relieve additional venous stasis.

The development of thrombus within tributary varicose veins is a common occurrence following phlebectomy procedures or microfoam ablation of the superficial axial veins. These patients have self-limited phlebitis induced by the procedure. Conservative treatment with non-steroidal anti-inflammatory medications and ice or heat should be employed in these cases. If symptomatic after 2–4 weeks, consider performing a stab microthrombectomy of the thrombosed superficial varicosities.

Clinical Practice Guidelines for the Treatment of SVT [17]

- SVT in the axial superficial veins and tributaries above the knee >3 cm from the junction with the deep veins and >5 cm in length: the recommendation is fondaparinux 2.5 mg subcutaneously daily for 45 days. Alternatively, rivaroxaban 10 mg orally daily for 45 days is an alternative. Recommendation 1 (strong) with Quality of Evidence A (high).
- Consensus statement: For patients with SVT in the axial superficial veins $\leq$3 cm from the saphenofemoral junction, treatment with full anticoagulation for a minimum of 6 weeks should be considered.
- For selected patients with isolated thrombosis of tributaries or limited involvement of the axial superficial veins, phlebectomy is a safe alternative once the pro-thrombotic period is over. Recommendation 2 (weak) and Quality of Evidence B (moderate).
- Consensus Statement: In patients with SVT, ablation should be performed once the inflammation has resolved, if there is evidence of pathologic reflux on duplex ultrasound.

Summary

Superficial vein thrombosis is no longer considered a benign entity. It carries a 25% chance of concurrent DVT, which may not be contiguous with the SVT, at the time of diagnosis. There is also a risk of thrombus extension, thrombus recurrence, and development of symptomatic DVT and PE over the ensuing three to twelve months.

Treatment with prophylactic or therapeutic doses of anticoagulation will depend on thrombus length, location, and risk stratification. Patients with SVT in the absence of varicose veins or superficial axial venous reflux should be considered for a hypercoagulable workup and screening for occult malignancy.

If superficial axial venous reflux is demonstrated on duplex ultrasound, consideration should be given to endovenous ablation procedures. This definitive treatment of underlying venous insufficiency may prevent SVT recurrence, which may occur in 10% to 20% of patients over time.

References

1. Bergqvist D, Jaroszewski H. Deep vein thrombosis in patients with superficial thrombophlebitis of the leg. Br Med J (Clin Res Ed). 1986;292(6521):658–9.
2. Chengelis DP, Bendick PJ, Glover JL, et al. Progression of superficial venous thrombosis to deep vein thrombosis. J Vasc Surg. 1996;24:745–9.
3. Frappe P, Buchmuller-Cordier A, Bertoletti L, et al. STEPH study group. Annual diagnosis rate of superficial vein thrombosis of the lower limbs: the STEPH community-based study. J Thromb Haemost. 2014;12:831–8.
4. Oger E. Incidence of venous thromboembolism: a community-based study in Western France. EPI-GETBO Study Group. Groupe d'Etude de la Thrombose de Bretagne Occidentale. Thromb Naemost. 2000;83:657–60.
5. Decousus H, Quere I, Presles E, et al. Superficial venous thrombosis and venous thromboembolism: a large, prospective epidemiologic study. Ann Intern Med. 2010;152(4):218–24.
6. Galanaud JP, Genty C, Sevestre MA, et al. Predictive factors for concurrent deep-vein thrombosis and symptomatic venous thromboembolic recurrence in care of superficial venous thrombosis. Thromb Haemost. 2011;105(1):31–9.
7. Decousus H, Bertoletti L, Frappe P. Spontaneous acute superficial vein thrombosis of the legs: do we really need to treat? J Thromb Haemost. 2015;13(Suppl 1):S230–7.
8. Verlato F, Zucchetta P, Prandoni P, et al. An unexpectedly high rate of pulmonary embolism in patients with superficial thrombophlebitis of the thigh. J Vasc Surg. 1999;30:1113–5.
9. IAC Standards and Guidelines for Vascular Testing Accreditation.
10. Mattos MA, Melendres G, Sumner DS, et al. Prevalence and distribution of calf vein thrombosis in patients with symptomatic deep venous thrombosis: a color-flow study. J Vasc Surg. 1996;24:738–44.
11. Aguilar C, del Villar V. D-dimer is not useful for the diagnosis of isolated superficial venous thrombosis. Am J Med. 2005;118:1417.e13–6.
12. Soyode E, Prichard W, Hayman M, et al. Validation of the age-adjusted D-dimer in an ambulatory deep vein thrombosis diagnostic service: beware of superficial thrombophlebitis. Br J Haematol. 2020;191:e94–6.

13. Decousus H, Prandoni P, Mismetti P, et al. Fondaparinux for the treatment of superficial-vein thrombosis in the legs. N Engl J Med. 2010;363:1222–32.
14. Beyer-Westendorf J, Schellong SM, Gerlach H, et al. Prevention of thromboembolic complications in patients with superficial-vein thrombosis given rivaroxaban or fondaparinux: the open-label, randomized, non-inferiority SURPRISE phase 3b trial. Lancet. 2017;4:e105–13.
15. Rabe E, Hoffmann U, Schimke A, et al. Determinants of late venous thromboembolic events after acute isolated superficial vein thrombosis in daily practice: 12 month results of the INSIGHTS-SVT study. Eur J Vasc Endovasc Surg. 2023;66:697–704.
16. Di Nisio M, Wichers IM, Middeldorp S, et al. Treatment for superficial thrombophlebitis of the leg. Cochrane Database Syst Rev. 2018;2:1–101.
17. Gloviczki P, Lawrence PF, Wasan SM, et al. The 2023 Society for Vascular Surgery, American Venous Forum, and American Vein and Lymphatic Society clinical practice guidelines for the management of varicose veins of the lower extremities. Part II. J Vasc Surg Venous Lymphat Disord. 2023:101670. (online ahead of print)
18. Husni EA, Williams WA. Superficial thrombophlebitis of lower limbs. Surgery. 1982;91:70–4.

Deep Vein Thrombosis

4

Carlos Echevarria and Gaurav Parmar

What can we learn about bears? Even in the absence of other health-related conditions, immobilization remains a significant risk factor for venous thromboembolism (VTE) … unless one is hibernating. A recent study described the risky task of collecting blood samples from 13 Swedish bears in their 4- to 7-month-long hibernation. The investigators discovered an antithrombotic key signature in the platelets of hibernating bears. Specifically, they identified that the downregulation of a heat shock protein, referred to as HSP47, causes a delay in the activation of the intrinsic pathway of coagulation. More importantly, they recognized the same pattern in healthy individuals after 27 days of voluntary immobilization, as well as chronically paralyzed patients [1]. This could

C. Echevarria (✉)
Division of Vascular and Endovascular Surgery, Department of Surgery, Massachusetts General Hospital/Harvard Venous & Lymphatic Medicine Alumni, Boston, MA, USA

Division of Vascular Medicine and Endovenous Interventions, Veins & Vascular Centers of Excellence, Phoenix, AZ, USA
e-mail: carlos.echevarria@vascular.md

G. Parmar
Vascular Medicine, Massachusetts General Hospital/Harvard Medical School, Boston, MA, USA
e-mail: GMParmar@mgh.harvard.edu

C. Echevarria et al. (eds.), *The Massachusetts General Hospital Protocols and Procedures for Venous Disease*,
https://doi.org/10.1007/978-3-032-05708-2_4

explain the low VTE risk in spinal cord injury patients, comparable to the general population [2–4].

Anatomy of the Disease

Despite being the number one cause of preventable death in the US, 1 in 4 people still die from conditions associated with thrombosis to this day [5]. To put this into perspective, VTE kills more people in any given year than breast cancer and prostate cancer combined [6, 7], and yet the level of awareness and prevention remains low. While the term "VTE" comprises a spectrum of diseases such as superficial venous thrombosis (SVT), pulmonary embolism (PE), and deep venous thrombosis (DVT), this chapter will focus specifically on DVT.

DVT can be classified as provoked or unprovoked. Those classified as provoked must have at least one acute risk factor triggering the event. Since such classification may have multiple ramifications and lifelong effects, detailed history taking is required, as chronic risk factors should not be considered an important contributor to an episode of acute DVT. Instead, include questions about recent conditions or situations that would be associated with sedentarism, ongoing pro-inflammatory processes, and the current list of medications.

Immobilization

Although surgeries and traumas are associated with an inflammatory response that may elicit thrombosis, prolonged immobilization is the common denominator in all cases [8, 9]. Studies from the early 2000s showed that up to 4–6% of high-risk subjects may develop DVT after long flights. These studies even concluded that mobility limitations in the non-aisle seats may increase the risk of developing DVT up to fourfold [10, 11]. With that said, it is very uncommon to develop a DVT just by sitting for an extended period of time. This supports the "multiple hit" hypothesis that additional risk factors play a role in the development of acute thrombus formation. In a population-based study, 89% of cases had at least one identifiable risk factor for thrombosis, with most having three or more [12].

Contraceptives and Other Medications

Estrogen-based oral contraceptives (OCPs) have been associated with an increased risk of DVT. However, the risk tends to decrease over time. In practice, the risk is the greatest in the first 3 months of use, but other risk-provoking factors should be evaluated if the patient is chronically on OCPs (>6–12 months) since the relative risk is halved. Only levonorgestrel-releasing intrauterine devices (IUD) and progesterone-only contraception have not been associated with increased thrombotic risk [13]. Other medications associated with increased risk of DVT include testosterone, tamoxifen, and corticosteroids.

Malignancies

One in five people with cancer will develop VTE [14]. While most cases of malignancy-associated VTE happen in known cancer cases, thrombosis could also be a harbinger of malignancy; 5–10% of idiopathic VTE cases may have a subsequent cancer diagnosis within 2 years [15–17]. The current recommendations are to complete age-appropriate cancer screening for all ages in those identified with acute DVT.

DVT Diagnosis

The clinical utility of individual signs or symptoms in DVT has been well studied. Homans' sign (calf pain with forced dorsiflexion of the affected limb) is unreliable at best. It has been observed more frequently in patients who displayed clinical signs of DVT but had negative venograms [18]. Furthermore, Homans' sign is positive in only one out of five necropsy-proven calf vein thromboses [19]. Any isolated sign or symptom is insufficient for diagnosis. However, the sensitivity and specificity dramatically increase when combined with a clinical pretest probability score, such as those used in the Well's criteria [20]. A Wells score ≤1 with a D-dimer within normal limits has been associated with a very low probability of DVT (mean 1.2%, 95% CI 0.7–1.8%), and as such, no further imaging is warranted [21].

DVT Treatment

- RE-COVER (2009): Dabigatran vs. warfarin in DVT
- RECORD1 (2009): Rivaroxaban vs. enoxaparin prophylaxis after hip surgery
- EINSTEIN-DVT (2010): Rivaroxaban vs. LMWH/warfarin in DVT
- EINSTEIN-PE (2012): Rivaroxaban in PE
- AMPLIFY (2013): Apixaban vs. LMWH/warfarin in DVT and PE
- AMPLIFY-EXT (2013): Apixaban for extended VTE treatment

Timeline of Anticoagulants [22]

Until 2009, warfarin (a vitamin K antagonist—VKA) was the standard of care for the treatment of VTE. However, the non-inferiority RE-COVER trial demonstrated that dabigatran, an oral direct thrombin inhibitor, was a good alternative with a 26% bleeding risk reduction compared to VKA [23]. This landmark study opened the gates for direct oral anticoagulants (DOACs) to become the mainstay of anticoagulation. Within the same year as RE-COVER, the RECORD1 trial demonstrated the effectiveness of rivaroxaban, an oral factor Xa inhibitor, in preventing VTE following hip orthopedic surgery [24]. After these findings, rivaroxaban expanded its use in DVT and PE treatments with the EINSTEIN trials (EINSTEIN-DVT 2010 and EINSTEIN-PE in 2012) [25, 26]. Apixaban, another oral factor Xa inhibitor, followed closely with

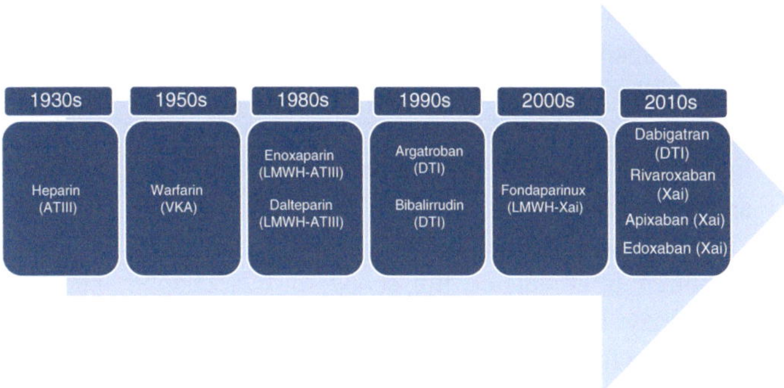

Fig. 4.1 Historic timeline of anticoagulants. ATIII: antithrombin III; VKA: vitamin K antagonist; LMWH: low molecular weight heparin; DTI: direct thrombin (IIa) inhibitor; Xai: direct factor Xa inhibitor

the AMPLIFY trial in 2013 [27]. Apixaban was found to have less clinically significant bleeding than conventional therapy as a composite outcome (4.3% vs. 9.7%; $p < 0.001$ for superiority; NNT 19). DOACs are now the recommended first-line therapy for the first 3 months after a DVT episode (see Fig. 4.1).

It is important to note that DOACs are contraindicated in the following conditions:

- Pregnancy/breastfeeding (this population was explicitly excluded from trials).
- Mechanical cardiac valves (warfarin remains the drug of choice. Future randomized controlled trials are necessary) [28].
- High-risk antiphospholipid syndrome.

Additional Considerations

Dosing

There is a tenfold higher rate of VTE recurrences if DOACs are given in a non-recommended dose or regimen [29]. The following are the recommended FDA-approved regimens for the treatment of DVT:

- Apixaban 10 mg BID for 7 days, then 5 mg twice daily[1]
- Rivaroxaban 15 mg BID for 3 weeks, then 20 mg daily
- Dabigatran 150 mg BID (after 5–10 days of parenteral anticoagulation—see Fig. 4.2)
- Edoxaban 60 mg QD (after 5–10 days of parenteral anticoagulation)[2]

Although it is outside the scope of this chapter, pediatric patients may be prescribed rivaroxaban and dabigatran in a weight-based fashion (Einstein-Jr).

Liver and Renal Failure

DOACs are not recommended for Child-Pugh class B or C (if you don't remember the scoring system, a simple way to think about it is that if the patient looks like a liver patient, they probably are class B already). LMWH is first-line therapy for end-stage liver disease.

DOACs for renal failure may require dose adjustments (see Table 4.1).

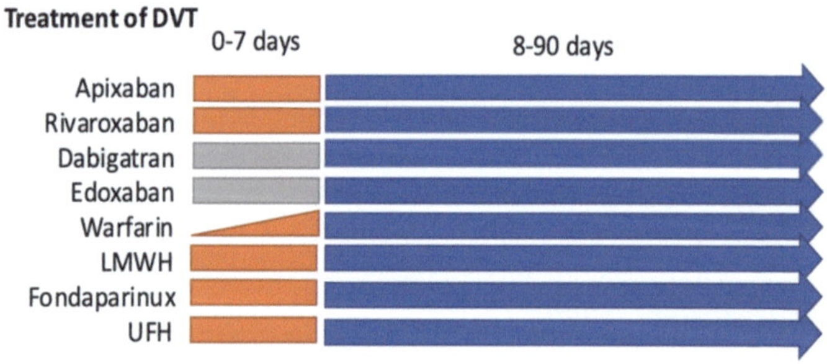

Fig. 4.2 Treatment of DVT. VKA, dabigatran, and edoxaban require parenteral agents for the first 5–10 days

[1] Dose reduction to 2.5 mg twice daily recommended for special population: age >80 years or body weight <60 kg.

[2] Dose reduction to 30 mg daily recommended for body weight <60 kg.

Table 4.1 DOAC dosing in renal failure based on creatine clearance

Cr Cl ml/min	>90	50-89	30-49	15-29	<15
Apixaban	5 mg BID	5 mg BID	5 mg BID	2.5 mg BID	2.5 mg BID[a]*
Rivaroxaban	20 mg QD	20 mg QD	15 mg QD	15 mg QD	Contraindicated
Dabigatran	150 mg BID	150 mg BID	75 mg BID	75 mg BID	Contraindicated
Edoxaban	60 mg QD	60 mg QD	30 mg QD	30 mg QD	Contraindicated

Color green: ok to use; yellow: dose adjustment/close monitoring; red: contraindicated

[a]FDA approved, but proceed with caution. The SAFE-HD trial and the AXADIA trial are ongoing to answer this question

Drug Interactions

Use caution when treating patients with medications that use the same CYP3A4 metabolic pathway since this can lead to varying DOAC metabolization (Table 4.2).

Choice of Anticoagulation

First-line therapy for anticoagulation is primarily determined by the underlying disease or clinical condition being treated. The choice of therapy should consider the patient's individual risks, comorbidities, and preferences, as well as any contraindications or potential drug interactions (Table 4.3).

Table 4.2 Conditions associated to CYP3A4 drug interaction (not a complete list)[a]

Anti-fungal, -virals, and antibiotics	Azoles, HIV meds, ciprofloxacin, erythro and clarithromycin, rifampin
Anti-inflammatories and pain	Steroids, fentanyl, methadone, colchicine
Cardiovascular medications	CCB, propranolol, clopidogrel, statins, cilostazol, sildenafil
Antihistamines and antacids	Cimetidine, astemizole, PPIs
Antiemetics	Ondansetron, aprepitant
Anxiety and sedation	Benzodiazepines, amitriptyline, trazodone, citalopram, buspirone
Antineoplastic agents	Multiple medications, including tamoxifen and finasteride
Anticonvulsants	Phenytoin, carbamazepine, oxcarbazepine
Immunosuppressive therapies	Sirolimus, tacrolimus
Psych and mood disorders	Quetiapine, risperidone, aripiprazole. Haloperidol

[a]For a more comprehensive list of medications, visit CYTOCHROME P450 DRUG INTERACTION TABLE (iu.edu)

Table 4.3 Anticoagulation selection based on background disease

Background	Preferred anticoagulant
End stage liver disease	LMWH
Renal disease Cr < 30 ml/min	VKA
History of gastrointestinal bleeding	VKA > apixaban > edoxaban > ribaroxaban
Coronary artery disease	VKA > DOACs (avoid dabigatran)
Cancer	LMWH > DOACs (use apixaban for GI malignancy)
Pregnancy	LMWH
Low platelet count (HIT)	Argatroban, bibalirudin, fondaparinux, DOACs
Mechanical heart valve	VKA (rivaroxaban needs further research)
Antiphospholipid syndrome	VKA

HIT heparin-induced thrombocytopenia, *VKA* vitamin K antagonist, *LMWH* low molecular weight heparin, *DOACs* direct oral anticoagulants

Special Populations

Obesity

Obesity has been shown to reduce CYP3A4 activity, potentially affecting DOACs metabolization. This results in increased substrate activity. However, more recent studies have validated the use of apixaban and rivaroxaban, regardless of patient BMI. Currently, there is insufficient data to support the use of dabigatran or edoxaban in this patient population [30].

Regarding bariatric surgery patients, there is more data to support the use of rivaroxaban than apixaban. However, due to malabsorption concerns, DOACs as a class are not recommended in the acute setting after a bariatric intervention. They may be considered 4 weeks after surgery. DOAC trough levels should be obtained to assess absorption and bioavailability [10].

DVT and Cancer

- CLOT (2003): LMWH vs. warfarin in cancer VTE
- SELECT-D (2018): Rivaroxaban vs. LMWH in cancer VTE
- Hokusai-VTE (2018): Edoxaban vs. LMWH in cancer VTE
- CARAVAGGIO (2020): Apixaban vs. dalteparin in cancer VTE
- ADAM VTE trial (2020): Apixaban vs. dalteparin in cancer VTE

Malignancy is the leading cause of VTE, with 20% of individuals with an underlying malignancy developing a VTE episode at any given time [14]. This risk has spearheaded a great interest in preventing malignancy-related VTE. In 2003, the CLOT trial found dalteparin superior to warfarin in preventing recurrent VTEs in those with known malignancies. Subsequently, multiple studies have evaluated DOACs, concluding that oral factor Xa inhibitors reduce the risk of recurrent VTE. However, edoxaban and rivaroxaban (SELECT-D and Hokusai-VTE) have shown a higher rate of gastrointestinal bleeding than LMWH. The CARAVAGGIO and ADAM VTE trial demonstrated the benefit of apixaban in cancer patients. Some have criticized that these studies included only a few patients with cancer of the upper gastrointestinal tract, limiting our interpretation of GI bleeding risk. All these studies excluded patients with metastases to the brain. Patients should consider wearing a medical bracelet with the DOAC they are taking; if clinically significant bleeding, the proper reversal agent can be administered more expeditiously.

In clinical practice, cancer-targeted and other pharmacologic therapies must be evaluated closely when selecting an anticoagulation strategy. DOACs are metabolized through the p-glycoprotein and CYP3A4 pathways, which can overlap with other pharmacologic therapies and affect their efficacy.

Location of DVT, Risk Factors, and Duration of Anticoagulation

The guidelines on DVT treatment are clear regardless of location, except for those below the knee. It is highly encouraged that vein specialists review their images. Relying on the report alone has led to overtreatment of below-knee DVTs. When encountering an episode of isolated below-knee thrombosis, one must consider symptoms. Although highly underutilized, monitoring with serial ultrasounds every 2 weeks is recommended for the asymptomatic patient [31]. Treatment is recommended in the event of thrombus extension or the development of symptoms. Duration of anticoagulation in VTE is dependent on provoking events and risk factors but also on the risk of recurrent VTE and bleeding risks. Recurrence rates are highest in the initial 3 months following the initial event. Recurrence rates for VTEs within the first year range from 10% to 15% for unprovoked VTEs and 1–5% for provoked VTEs. The annual recurrence risk of VTEs decreases after the first year. Bleeding risks increase with factors such as age, malignancy, hepatic or renal dysfunction, and anemia. For low-risk patients (0 risk factors), the total annual risk of significant bleeding is 0.8%, while those in a

Table 4.4 Risk factors for bleeding with anticoagulation therapy

Age >65	Metastatic cancer	History of bleeding
Age >75	Diabetes	History of stroke
Alcohol	Fall risk	Reduced functional capacity
Anemia	Liver failure	Recent surgery
Antiplatelet therapy	Subtherapeutic anticoagulation	Renal failure
Cancer		Thrombocytopenia

high-risk category (two or more risk factors) have a ≥6.5% annual risk of major bleeding. Risk factors for bleeding with anticoagulant therapy are detailed below (see Table 4.4).

The recommended duration of anticoagulation therapy for the first episode of a provoked proximal DVT is 3 months. In unprovoked proximal DVT, extended anticoagulation is recommended for those at low or moderate bleeding risk. However, for those at high bleeding risk, 3 months of therapy can be considered [32].

Endovascular and Surgical Interventions

- CAVENT trial (2012): PTS after CDT in iliofemoral vein thrombosis
- ATTRACT trial (2016): PTS after CDT in iliofemoral vein thrombosis

The treatment for acute DVT depends on two major factors: the location of the DVT and the bleeding risk. In the CAVENT trial, evaluating catheter-directed thrombolysis (CDT) versus anticoagulation in DVTs, the findings supported the use of CDT in iliofemoral DVTs by reducing the incidence of post-thrombotic syndrome (PTS) at 2 years. The ATTRACT trial did not support these findings. The incidence of PTS was not statistically significantly different in either arm. However, a subgroup analysis in the CDT arm suggested a modest reduction in severe PTS symptoms (18% vs. 24%; $p = 0.04$). Variations of the pharmacomechanical method of thrombolysis and loss of follow-up in a significant proportion of patients in the control group might have underestimated the treatment effect. We discuss this topic further in the deep venous insufficiency chapter.

Perioperative Management of Anticoagulation [33]

Perioperative management of anticoagulation requires a fine balance between keeping the risk of DVT at bay and decreasing the risk of bleeding to a minimum. Those at high risk for recurrent VTE include those with a recent episode of thrombosis within the last 3 months, a history of thrombophilia, or active malignancies. The degree of limited mobility in the postoperative period will add to the risk of thrombosis.

In the era of DOACs, surgical bleeding risks must also be considered for perioperative anticoagulation management. Surgeries with higher bleeding risk, such as major orthopedic surgeries, cancer surgeries including solid tumor resections, and cardiac surgeries, should consider earlier interruption of anticoagulation and resumption after 48–72 h postoperatively. The table below graphically represents the various strategies for DOACs in the perioperative period (Fig. 4.3).

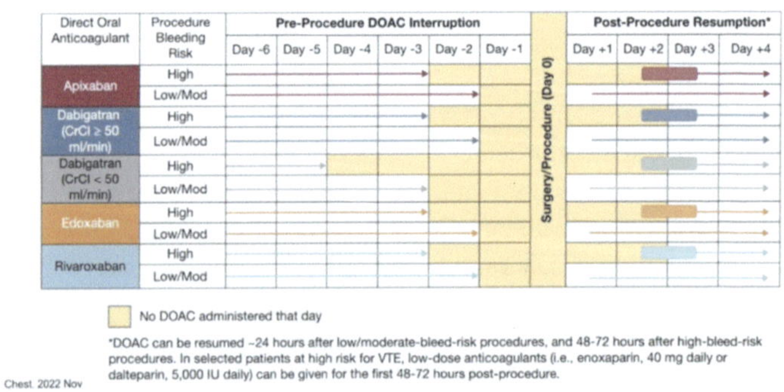

Fig. 4.3 Peri-operative management. Low to moderate-bleeding risk surgeries require only 24 h of DOAC discontinuation prior to the procedure, compared to 48 h for high-bleeding risk cases, except for dabigatran (discontinue 96 h prior to intervention). (CHEST guidelines - Elsevier with granted permission [33])

For warfarin, a similar strategy can be utilized. Warfarin should be discontinued 5 days before a procedure and resumed on the evening of the procedure. Bridging with heparin products is no longer recommended in patients receiving warfarin, except for those at high risk of VTE. Bridging is generally *not* suggested for patients with arrhythmias, mechanical heart valves, or low to moderate risk of VTE, due to evidence showing no significant reduction in thromboembolic events but a significant increase in major bleeding risk. Bridging may be considered in selective high-risk patients, such as those with a recent stroke (<3 months), recent transient ischemic attacks, or acute VTE (<3 months), severe thrombophilia, active cancer with high-risk VTE features, or mechanical mitral valves *with* additional stroke risk factors [33].

Evaluating for Thrombophilias

The contemporary concept of thrombophilia originated in the mid-20th century, evolving from a rare familial condition to a set of identifiable risk factors, thanks to the discovery of specific genetic mutations and protein deficiencies. With no further major recent discoveries, this puts into perspective how little we know about unprovoked thrombosis (Fig. 4.4). Testing for heritable thrombophilia should only be considered in select patients

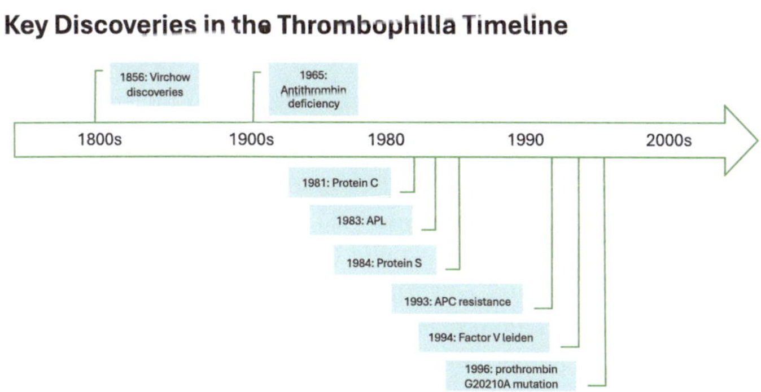

Fig. 4.4 Thrombophilia timeline. *APL* antiphospholipid syndrome, *APC* activated protein C resistance

with VTEs because testing in all cases does not translate into a decreased risk of VTE recurrence [34]. Contemplate testing in individuals with early VTEs (before the age of 40) or with a strong family history of VTEs (more than two family members with thrombotic episodes or family history of thrombophilia) [35].

Duration of anticoagulation is not dependent on an underlying thrombophilia; rather, as detailed previously, the duration depends on whether the DVT was provoked or unprovoked and the risk of bleeding with anticoagulation therapy. The same goes for the choice of anticoagulation therapy, with one particular exception: antiphospholipid syndrome (APS). Patients with arterial APS or Triple-positive antiphospholipid syndrome (TPAPS) require VKA as first-line therapy. TPAPS refers to a diagnosis where a patient tests positive for all three types of antiphospholipid antibodies: lupus anticoagulant (LA), anti-beta-2-glycoprotein I (B2GPI), and anticardiolipin antibodies (aCL).

Pregnancy and VTE

There is an up to five times increase in risk of VTE during pregnancy or puerperium. That risk is increased hundredfold if there is a personal history of VTE. Therefore, all women should be evaluated for risk factors for VTE. Aside from the common risk factors such as prolonged immobility, venous varicosities, thrombophilias, or proinflammatory disorders, some pregnancy-related risk factors need to be considered (Table 4.5).

If a woman of childbearing age has a history of prior unprovoked VTE, they should be screened for inherited or acquired thrombophilia. These individuals should also be considered for postpartum low molecular weight heparin. If a woman has a history of recurrent VTEs or has had an episode of thrombophilia-related VTE, low molecular weight heparin should be considered in the antenatal period and for at least 6 weeks postpartum. A summary of the recommendations for thromboprophylaxis in pregnancy and puerperium is included below (Fig. 4.5).

Table 4.5 Risk factors for thrombosis in pregnancy and puerperium

Pregnancy	Peripartum
Age >35 or parity >3	Prolonged labor
Multiple pregnancy or ART	Excessive blood loss
Initial obesity (BMI > 30 kg/m^2)	Mid-cavity instrumental delivery
Hyperemesis gravida or dehydration	Peripartum surgical procedure (e.g. ERPC or cesarian)
Pre-eclampsia	Postpartum infection

ART assisted reproductive technology (e.g., IVF), *ERPC* evacuation of retained products of conception

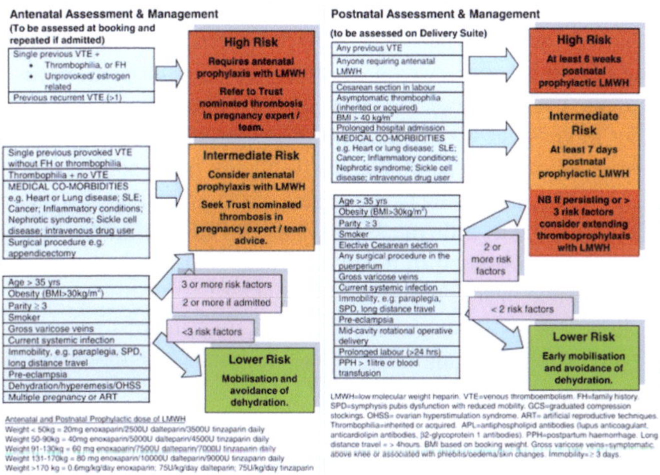

Fig. 4.5 Obstetric thromboprophylaxis risk assessment and management [36]

Hospitalized Individuals and VTE Risk

There is more than a hundred times greater risk of developing a VTE when an individual is hospitalized with an acute illness compared to the general population [37]. VTE risk assessment scores, such as the Padua Prediction Scoring System, IMPROVE model, and Caprini Score, are all commonly used risk assessment tools that can help stratify patients for consideration of prophylactic therapy in hospitalized medical patients. Although they slightly differ in their design and application, the Padua and IMPROVE models primarily focus on identifying patients at high risk for VTE by evaluating factors such as age, immobility, history of cancer, and prior history of VTE. They are widely used due to their simplicity and have been externally validated in various settings. The Caprini Score, which is most often applied in surgical patients, evaluates risk based on factors similar to those of the other models but with a more detailed scoring system stratifying risk based on the type of surgery. While all three models aim to identify high-risk patients, the choice of tool often depends on the clinical context, with the Padua and IMPROVE models being more commonly used in medical patients and the Caprini Score often favored in surgical settings (Table 4.6).

Low-risk patients generally do not require pharmacologic prophylaxis; early ambulation and mechanical methods can be utilized.

Table 4.6 Comparative analysis outlining key aspects of VTE risk scores in hospitalized patients

Padua prediction scoring system (medical patients)	IMPROVE model[a] (medical patients)	Caprini score (surgical patients)
Age > 70 years	Age > 60 years	Age (stratified by age range)
History of VTE	History of VTE	Recent (<1 m) medical history
Reduced mobility	Reduced mobility	Venous disease or clotting disorder
Active cancer	Active cancer	Reduced mobility

(continued)

Table 4.6 (continued)

Padua prediction scoring system (medical patients)	IMPROVE model[a] (medical patients)	Caprini score (surgical patients)
Thrombophilia	Thrombophilia	Acute and chronic medical conditions (e.g., obesity, heart failure, diabetes)
Recent surgery or trauma	ICU/CCU stay	
Acute and chronic medical conditions (e.g. obesity, MI, CVA)		
Hormonal treatment		

[a]The IMPROVEDD model includes D-dimer ≥2× ULN

Surveillance Recommendations After DVT

- *PROLONG* (2006): D-Dimer testing after VTE
- *AMPLIFY-EXT* (2013): Apixaban after VTE treatment
- *ASPIRE* (2012): Aspirin after VTE treatment
- *AMPLIFY-EXT* (2013): Apixaban for extended VTE prophylaxis
- *EINSTEIN CHOICE* (2017): Rivaroxaban vs. aspirin for extended VTE prophylaxis
- *DODS* (2019): D-dimer based anticoagulation discontinuation

The rate of VTE recurrence is up to 11% in the first year alone, prompting investigators to study additional methods to avoid recurrent episodes. An early trial from 2006 showed that a positive D-dimer at 4 weeks after discontinuation of oral anticoagulation after acute VTE increased the risk of recurrent DVT (HR 4.26). This suggested that using a D-dimer for surveillance may help determine who should be restarted on oral anticoagulation. The DODS trial attempted to assess this concept again for unprovoked DVTs and found that, although female patients could benefit from D-dimer risk stratification, the 7.5% rate of recurrence in (−) D-dimer male patients questioned the benefits of this method.

Pharmacological methods were first assessed with the ASPIRE and WARFASA trials (2012), demonstrating that aspirin reduces VTE recurrence by 32%, while AMPLIFY-EXT studied apixaban, a factor Xa inhibitor. AMPLIFY-EXT (an extension of the 2013 AMPLIFY trial) randomized 2482 patients with VTE who have completed 6–12 months of anticoagulation to apixaban 2.5 mg bid, apixaban 5 mg bid, or matching placebo. Compared to placebo, the low and high doses of apixaban were associated with 63% and 67% reductions in the primary endpoint of recurrent VTE or all-cause mortality. Neither dose of apixaban increased the rate of significant bleeding. The 2017 EINSTEIN CHOICE trial has also studied rivaroxaban's use for prolonged VTE treatment. Recurrent VTE occurred at a rate of 1.2% in patients receiving rivaroxaban 10 mg/d qd vs. 4.4% in those with low-dose aspirin.

Lifetime anticoagulation must consider the risks and benefits of treatment and encompass laboratory findings and an individualized patient assessment. Shared decision-making promotes patients' active participation in their care.

Summary

Venous thromboembolism (VTE) kills more people in any given year than breast cancer and prostate cancer combined, and yet the level of awareness and prevention remains low. Conditions like obesity, malignancies, the use of contraceptives, or immobilization can increase thrombosis risk. That said, it is very uncommon to develop a VTE just by sitting for an extended period. This supports the "multiple hit" hypothesis that additional risk factors play a role in developing acute thrombus formation. The advent of direct oral anticoagulants has simplified the treatment of acute thrombosis. Still, this statement cannot be applied as an absolute, as conditions such as renal or liver failure and special populations require dose adjustments or alternative treatments.

References

1. Thienel M, Müller-Reif J, et al. Immobility-associated thromboprotection is conserved across mammalian species from bear to human. Science. 2023;380:178–87.
2. Godat LN, Kobayashi L, Chang DC, Coimbra R. Can we ever stop worrying about venous thromboembolism after trauma? J Trauma Acute Care Surg. 2015;78:475–81.
3. Giorgi Pierfranceschi M, et al. The short- and long-term risk of venous thromboembolism in patients with acute spinal cord injury: a prospective cohort study. Thromb Haemost. 2013;109:34–8.
4. Maxwell RA, et al. Routine prophylactic vena cava filtration is not indicated after acute spinal cord injury. J Trauma. 2002;52:902–6.
5. Lozano R, Naghavi M, Foreman K, et al. Global and regional mortality from 235 causes of death for 20 age groups in 1990 and 2010: a systematic analysis for the Global Burden of Disease Study 2010. Lancet. 2012;380:2095–128. https://doi.org/10.1016/S0140-6736(12)61728-0.
6. https://gis.cdc.gov/Cancer/USCS/#/Trends/.
7. Beckman MG, Hooper WC, Critchley SE, Ortel TL. Venous thromboembolism: a public health concern. Am J Prev Med. 2010;38(4 Suppl):S495–501. https://doi.org/10.1016/j.amepre.2009.12.017. PMID: 20331949.
8. Stark K, Massberg S. Interplay between inflammation and thrombosis in cardiovascular pathology. Nat Rev Cardiol. 2021;18(9):666–82. https://doi.org/10.1038/s41569-021-00552-1. Epub 2021 May 6. PMID: 33958774; PMCID: PMC8100938.
9. Mula V, Parikh S, Suresh S, et al. Venous thromboembolism rates after hip and knee arthroplasty and hip fractures. BMC Musculoskelet Disord. 2020;21:95. https://doi.org/10.1186/s12891-020-3100-4.
10. Belcaro G, et al. Venous thromboembolism from air travel: the LONFLIT study. Angiology. 2001;52:369–74.
11. Cesarone MR, et al. Venous thrombosis from air travel: the LONFLIT3 study prevention with aspirin vs low-molecular-weight heparin (LMWH) in high-risk subjects: a randomized trial. Angiology. 2002;53:1–6.
12. Spencer FA, Emery C, Lessard D, Anderson F, Emani S, Aragam J, Becker RC, Goldberg RJ. The Worcester Venous Thromboembolism study: a population-based study of the clinical epidemiology of venous thromboembolism. J Gen Intern Med. 2006;21(7):722–7. https://doi.org/10.1111/j.1525-1497.2006.00458.x. PMID: 16808773; PMCID: PMC1924694.
13. Keenan L, Kerr T, Duane M, Van Gundy K. Systematic review of hormonal contraception and risk of venous thrombosis. Linacre Q. 2018;85(4):470–7. https://doi.org/10.1177/0024363918816683. Epub 2019 Jan 3. PMID: 32431379; PMCID: PMC6322116.

14. Mulder FI, Horváth-Puhó E, van Es N, van Laarhoven HWM, Pedersen L, Moik F, Ay C, Büller HR, Sørensen HT. Venous thromboembolism in cancer patients: a population-based cohort study. Blood. 2021;137(14):1959–69. https://doi.org/10.1182/blood.2020007338. PMID: 33171494.
15. Sørensen HT, Mellemkjaer L, Steffensen FH, Olsen JH, Nielsen GL. The risk of a diagnosis of cancer after primary deep venous thrombosis or pulmonary embolism. N Engl J Med. 1998;338(17):1169–73.
16. Chung WS, Lin CL, Hsu WH, Sung FC, Li RY, Kao CH. Idiopathic venous thromboembolism: a potential surrogate for occult cancer. QJM. 2014;107(7):529–36. https://doi.org/10.1093/qjmed/hcu023. Epub 2014 Jan 27. PMID: 24472734.
17. Carrier M, Le Gal G, Wells PS, Fergusson D, Ramsay T, Rodger MA. Systematic review: the Trousseau syndrome revisited: should we screen extensively for cancer in patients with venous thromboembolism? Ann Intern Med. 2008;149(5):323–33. https://doi.org/10.7326/0003-4819-149-5-200809020-00007. PMID: 18765702.
18. O'Donnel TF Jr, et al. Diagnosis of deep venous thrombosis in the outpatient by venography. Surg Gynecol Obstet. 1980;150(1):69–74.
19. McLachlin J, et al. An evaluation of clinical signs in the diagnosis of venous thrombosis. Arch Surg. 1962;85:58–65.
20. Modi S, et al. Wells criteria for DVT is a reliable clinical tool to assess the risk of deep venous thrombosis in trauma patients. World J Emerg Surg. 2016;11:24.
21. Geersing GJ, et al. Exclusion of deep vein thrombosis using the Wells rule in clinically important subgroups: individual patient data meta-analysis. BMJ. 2014;348:g1340.
22. Montinari MR, et al. Eighty years of oral anticoagulation: learning from history. Vasc Pharmacol. 2021;141:106918.
23. Schulman S, et al. Dabigatran versus warfarin in the treatment of acute venous thromboembolism. N Engl J Med. 2009;361(24):2342–52.
24. Eriksson BI, et al. Rivaroxaban versus enoxaparin for thromboprophylaxis after hip arthroplasty. N Engl J Med. 2008;358(26):2765–75.
25. Bauersachs R, et al. Oral rivaroxaban for symptomatic venous thromboembolism. N Engl J Med. 2010;363(26):2499–510.
26. Büller HR, et al. Oral rivaroxaban for the treatment of symptomatic pulmonary embolism. N Engl J Med. 2012;366(14):1287–97.
27. Agnelli G, et al. Oral apixaban for the treatment of acute venous thromboembolism. N Engl J Med. 2013;369(9):799–808.
28. Ryu R, Tran R. DOACs in mechanical and bioprosthetic heart valves: a narrative review of emerging data and future directions. Clin Appl Thromb Hemost. 2022;28:10760296221103578. https://doi.org/10.1177/10760296221103578.

29. Trujillo-Santos J, Di Micco P, Dentali F, Douketis J, Díaz-Peromingo JA, Núñez MJ, Cañas I, Mastroiacovo D, Saraiva de Sousa M, Monreal M, RIETE Investigators. Real-life treatment of venous thromboembolism with direct oral anticoagulants: the influence of recommended dosing and regimens. Thromb Haemost. 2017;117(2):382–9. https://doi.org/10.1160/TH16-07-0494. Epub 2016 Oct 27. PMID: 27786333.
30. Martin K, et al. Use of direct oral anticoagulants in patients with obesity for treatment and prevention of venous thromboembolism: updated communication from the ISTH SSC Subcommittee on Control of Anticoagulation. J Thromb Haemost. 2021;19(8):1874–82.
31. Fleck D, Albadawi H, Wallace A, Knuttinen G, Naidu S, Oklu R. Below-knee deep vein thrombosis (DVT): diagnostic and treatment patterns. Cardiovasc Diagn Ther. 2017;7(Suppl 3):S134–9. https://doi.org/10.21037/cdt.2017.11.03. PMID: 29399516; PMCID: PMC5778527.
32. Kearon C, Akl EA, Comerota AJ, Prandoni P, Bounameaux H, Goldhaber SZ, Nelson ME, Wells PS, Gould MK, Dentali F, Crowther M, Kahn SR. Antithrombotic therapy for VTE disease: Antithrombotic Therapy and Prevention of Thrombosis, 9th ed: American College of Chest Physicians Evidence-Based Clinical Practice Guidelines. Chest. 2012;141(2 Suppl):e419S–96S. https://doi.org/10.1378/chest.11-2301. Erratum in: Chest. 2012;142(6):1698–704. PMID: 22315268; PMCID: PMC3278049.
33. Douketis JD, et al. Perioperative management of antithrombotic therapy: an American College of Chest Physicians Clinical Practice Guideline. Chest. 2022;162(5):e207–43.
34. Coppens M, Reijnders JH, Middeldorp S, Doggen CJM, Rosendaal FR. Testing for inherited thrombophilia does not reduce the recurrence of venous thrombosis. J Thromb Haemost. 2008;6(9):1474–7. https://doi.org/10.1111/j.1538-7836.2008.03055.x.
35. Baglin T, Gray E, Greaves M, Hunt BJ, Keeling D, Machin S, Mackie I, Makris M, Nokes T, Perry D, Tait RC, Walker I, Watson H, British Committee for Standards in Haematology. Clinical guidelines for testing for heritable thrombophilia. Br J Haematol. 2010;149(2):209–20. https://doi.org/10.1111/j.1365-2141.2009.08022.x. Epub 2010 Jan 28. PMID: 20128794.
36. Frise CJ, MacCallum PK, Mackillop LH, Based on Royal College of Obstetricians and Gynaecologists, et al. Thromboprophylaxis during pregnancy, labour and after vaginal delivery. RCOG guideline no. 37. London: Royal College of Obstetricians and Gynaecologists; 2004.
37. Heit JA, Melton LJ 3rd, Lohse CM, Petterson TM, Silverstein MD, Mohr DN, O'Fallon WM. Incidence of venous thromboembolism in hospitalized patients vs community residents. Mayo Clin Proc. 2001;76(11):1102–10. https://doi.org/10.4065/76.11.1102. PMID: 11702898.

Part III

Arterial Considerations for the Vein Specialist

The Great Saphenous Vein as a Conduit

5

Syed Moez Shah Bukhari, Syed T. Ahsan, Gloria Salazar, and Luis Suarez

Special Considerations Regarding Treatment of the Saphenous Vein

The surgical treatment of the saphenous vein is one of the most performed procedures for managing peripheral venous insufficiency and its complications. In patients presenting with symptomatic varicose veins with pain, edema, or wounds and evidence of valvular reflux of more than 0.5 s on duplex ultrasound, treatment is indicated.

S. M. S. Bukhari
Department of Cardiovascular Disease, Johns Hopkins University, Baltimore, MD, USA
e-mail: sbukhar3@jh.edu

Syed T. Ahsan
Division of Vascular Medicine Henry Ford Hospital, Detroit, MI, USA
e-mail: sahsan4@hfhs.org

G. Salazar
Department of Radiology, University of North Carolina at Chapel Hill, Chapel Hill, NC, USA
e-mail: gloria_salazar@med.unc.edu

L. Suarez (✉)
Division of Vascular and Endovascular Surgery Department of Surgery, Massachusetts General Hospital/Harvard Medical School, Boston, MA, USA
e-mail: Lsuarez7@mgh.harvard.edu

C. Echevarria et al. (eds.), *The Massachusetts General Hospital Protocols and Procedures for Venous Disease*,
https://doi.org/10.1007/978-3-032-05708-2_5

Treatment aims to interrupt the venous reflux, either by ligating and stripping the vein or, more recently, with minimally invasive techniques like thermal or non-thermal ablation.

According to the most recent American Venous Forum (AVF) guidelines for the management of varicose veins, there is no established strict diameter of the great saphenous vein (GSV) to consider when treating if the severity of the symptoms justifies intervention [1]. However, in a subset of patients with a higher cardiovascular risk, the GSV (and, to a lesser extent, the SSV) could be used as a conduit for surgical bypass interventions, and consideration should be given to preserving the GSV in these patients.

The Saphenous Vein

The ideal saphenous vein to use for a bypass should measure >2.5 mm in diameter with sufficient length to reach from the origin or inflow of the bypass to the target or outflow; this length requires even greater consideration when used for lower extremity distal bypasses.

The vein should be patent and compressible when evaluated on a grayscale ultrasound, with normal wall thickness and minimal tortuosity during surgical exploration. Although there is no consensus on graft cut-off size, saphenous veins ≥6 mm are less frequently used due to the risk of compliance mismatch (leading to complications such as intimal hyperplasia and graft failure), poor endothelial regeneration, and increased risk of graft aneurysmal dilation [2–4].

For most applications, saphenous vein grafts have better patency than the prosthetic alternatives and are more resistant to infection. For this reason, saphenous veins are recommended for use in contaminated or infected fields and trauma.

Patients at Risk

The population at risk of revascularization with a vein conduit is a similar age group with significant cardiovascular risk factors; this includes age >65, smoking, diabetes, hypertension, chronic kidney disease, hyperlipidemia, or any previous interventions for coronary artery disease or peripheral vascular disease. These conditions lead to atherosclerosis and, eventually, stenosis in multiple arterial trees. This applies to the lower extremities, as well as cardiovascular, neurovascular, and mesenteric circulation.

Peripheral Arterial Disease (PAD): The Debate

- BEST CLI trial (2022): Bypass surgery vs. endovascular
- Contextualizing the BEST-CLI Trial (2023)
- FOURIER Trial (2018): PCSK9 Inhibition for LDL-C
- VOYAGER PAD trial (2020): Rivaroxaban in PAD

Luis Suarez, Vascular Surgery Perspective

Millions around the world are affected by lower extremity peripheral arterial disease (PAD), with the most severe cases leading to chronic pain and amputation. Symptoms can range from mild claudication to critical limb ischemia and tissue loss, ranging from toe ulcers to gangrene.

With the advent of endovascular minimally invasive therapies, most patients are treated by endovascular means, either with angioplasty or stenting. However, multiple trials failed to prove a difference in outcomes against traditional open-vein bypass surgery. This was until recently when the BEST CLI trial was published [5]. This was a prospective multicenter randomized multidisciplinary trial. Two cohorts were created with the recruited patients: those with available single-segment saphenous veins (Cohort 1) and those without (Cohort 2). One thousand four hundred sixty-seven patients were recruited in Cohort 1 and randomized for endovascular first treatment vs. bypass. Those patients who received a vein bypass had significantly lower Major Adverse Limb Events (MALE) compared to the endovascular arm, 42.6% vs. 57.4%, respectively (hazard ratio, 0.68; 95% confidence interval [CI], 0.59 to 0.79; $p < 0.001$). This was secondary to a lower amputation rate in the surgical arm and a higher reintervention rate in the endovascular arm. Mortality was similar between both groups.

Saphenous vein preservation should be considered in patients with venous disease at high risk for PAD, as it may become a usable conduit for bypass in the future with great benefits for this population.

This information can be extrapolated to patients in need of an upper extremity arterial bypass. Upper extremity arterial disease is less frequent. In patients with supraclavicular disease, the use of prosthetic bypass is accepted, as the patency of these shorter bypasses is equivalent to those with veins, and the location of the graft benefits from the stiffness and protection offered by ring ePTFE grafts. For below-the-clavicle disease, vein bypasses are indicated, and the lower extremity saphenous vein remains the preferred conduit.

Gloria Salazar, Interventional Radiology Perspective

With the advent of catheter-based techniques, endovascular treatment for PAD has gained significant traction, given the potential for fewer complications and cost savings compared to surgical approaches. However, recent literature with the BEST-CLI publication has challenged this rationale. It is essential to highlight that in this trial, patients enrolled were predominantly white (72%). Additionally, they were younger (66.9 ± 9.9 SD), less gender diverse (28.5% females), and with fewer comorbidities than those resembling the Medicare population, in which chronic limb-threatening ischemia (CLTI) is very prevalent. PAD disparities are well known, with a higher proportion of African American and Hispanic patients undergoing amputation [6]. The lack of diversity in clinical trials evaluating endovascular therapies limits the generalizability of study results for clinical application, leading to uncertainty in health outcomes.

To test the external validity of the BEST CLI trial, a recent study evaluated the same eligibility for interventions and outcomes in a more gender-diverse group of Medicare patients with older age and more comorbidities [7]. In addition, this observational study illustrated the diversity of treatment and treating physicians. While surgical alternatives for PAD patients are only within the vascular surgeons' scope of practice, endovascular therapies can be performed by interventional radiologists, cardiologists, and vascular surgeons alike, and differences in procedural choice may influence patient outcomes. Endovascular operators for the Medicare population study were less likely to be surgeons (55.9% [26,924/48,148] vs. 73.0% [520/708]) and more likely to be cardiologists (25.5% [5900/48,148] vs. 14.5% [103/78]).

The Medicare population observational study demonstrated that surgical and endovascular revascularization outcomes differ from the BEST CLI trial, with a higher cumulative incidence of adverse events in patients treated with surgical approaches (irrespective of autologous or non-autologous grafts). Additionally, the study showed less than half the frequency of major reinterventions for endovascular procedures than those observed in the BEST-CLI trial (technical failures were not captured in the data analysis). Even with the limitations inherent in this observational study, the analysis highlights the need to further understand the context in which treating physicians are practicing and the application of controlled study results to real-world patient populations.

Syed Bukhari & Syed Ahsan, Cardiology/Vascular Medicine Perspective

Although data from randomized controlled trials and real-world studies show differing outcomes when comparing surgical and endovascular interventions, both approaches provide unique opportunities for personalized treatment strategies based on selected patient characteristics and individual treatment goals. Patient-specific factors, including lesion anatomy, conduit availability, and comorbidity burden, may influence the choice of the optimal revascularization strategy. Long-segment lesions affecting below-knee popliteal and infra-popliteal arteries may be better suited for surgical intervention. In contrast, the lack of a suitable autogenous vein or high perioperative risk due to comorbidities may make endovascular revascularization preferable. Additionally, incorporating patient preferences through shared decision-making remains a crucial aspect of treatment planning.

Despite significant progress in the interventional space, optimal medical management—focused on controlling cardiovascular risk factors such as hypertension, diabetes mellitus, and lipid abnormalities, coupled with the adoption of a healthy lifestyle that includes exercise, balanced nutrition, and smoking cessation—remains fundamental to PAD management. In patients requiring endovascular or surgical intervention, ongoing adherence to optimal medical therapy improves functional outcomes and reduces post-interventional mortality [8, 9]. The addition of promising new treatments to the therapeutic armamentarium for PAD has expanded options for effective management and better outcomes, especially in the advanced stages of the disease.

One such advancement is evolocumab, a proprotein convertase subtilisin–kexin type 9 (PCSK9) inhibitor, which is now included in the most recent 2024 ACC/AHA PAD guidelines as an adjunct to high-intensity statins to achieve a low-density lipoprotein cholesterol (LDL-C) level of <70 mg/dL. The FOURIER trial, which evaluated evolocumab in over 3600 PAD patients, demonstrated a significant reduction in median LDL-C by approximately 30 mg/dL, along with a decrease in major adverse cardiovascular events (MACE) (HR 0.73, 95% CI 0.59, 0.91) and major adverse limb events (MALE) (HR 0.58, 95% CI 0.38, 0.88). Most notably, intensive LDL-C lowering with evolocumab resulted in greater absolute risk reductions in MACE and MALE in individuals with chronic limb-threatening ischemia compared to those with intermittent claudication, underscoring the potential benefits of aggressive medical management for high-risk individuals [10].

Antiplatelet and antithrombotic therapies are crucial components of PAD management. While the role of aspirin monotherapy in PAD has long been established, the VOYAGER PAD trial evaluated a regimen of low-dose rivaroxaban (2.5 mg twice daily) in addition to low-dose aspirin in patients following lower extremity revascularization [11]. This combination significantly reduced the risk of MACE and MALE, primarily through lower rates of acute limb ischemia. As a result, the most recent PAD guidelines recommend the dual antithrombotic regimen of aspirin and low-dose rivaroxaban as a Class I indication (level of evidence A) for patients who have undergone endovascular or surgical revascularization.

Finally, the emergence of sodium-glucose transporter-2 (SGLT-2) inhibitors and glucagon-like peptide-1 (GLP-1) agonists in the therapeutic landscape has provided benefits beyond diabetes control. These medications have demonstrated a significant reduction in MACE in patients with type 2 diabetes mellitus, a substantial proportion of whom had concomitant PAD, thereby establishing their role as part of guideline-directed therapies for PAD.

In summary, while current data does not conclusively establish the superiority of one revascularization strategy over another, patient-specific factors and preferences may guide the decision-making process. Significantly, this ongoing debate over the optimal revascularization approach should not overshadow the imperative of implementing optimal, guideline-directed medical therapies, which are equally vital in preventing adverse outcomes.

Coronary Artery Bypass Graft (CABG)

Patients with significant coronary artery disease (CAD) present with symptoms ranging from mild exertional dyspnea, stable chronic angina, and unstable angina to acute myocardial infarction. When indicated, these are mostly treated with percutaneous coronary intervention (PCI) because of the minimally invasive nature with lower morbidity and mortality. Still, randomized trials have shown the superiority of CABG over PCI in patients with higher disease burden and lesion complexity [12] and diabetic patients [13]. Specifically, left main coronary artery disease, diffuse three-vessel coronary disease with >70% stenosis, and multivessel disease with diabetes or left ventricular dysfunction are more amenable to CABG procedures [8, 10]. A Saphenous Vein Graft (SVG) may still be needed in these patients.

The preferred graft for coronary artery bypass is arterial conduits like the internal mammary artery or harvested radial artery. However, if this is not available or in patients with multi-vessel disease, saphenous vein graft is indicated.

The characteristics of the saphenous conduit are similar to those of patients with lower extremity disease, but a shorter length is usually needed.

Mesenteric Ischemia

Mesenteric ischemia occurs secondary to the interruption of blood flow to the intestine, leading to mucosal damage, progressing to transmural necrosis, and, if untreated, death. This can present acutely or chronically, depending on the timing of symptoms.

Acute mesenteric ischemia (AMI) occurs suddenly and could be secondary to occlusive (embolism or thrombosis) or non-occlusive (NOMI) secondary to global hypoperfusion through previous stenosis. Commonly presents with acute onset of poorly localized abdominal pain that is out of proportion to physical exam findings; when presenting with peritonitis symptoms, bowel perforation should be suspected. Chronic mesenteric ischemia (CMI) presentation is more insidious and usually presents with a classic triad of symptoms with postprandial abdominal pain, weight loss, and food fear. However, it is imperative to note that this triad is not always present, even at the time of revascularization, and patients can present with nonspecific intestinal complaints, including abdominal discomfort, nausea/vomiting, diarrhea, and constipation [14].

In patients with CMI, when treatment is indicated, the main target for revascularization should be the superior mesenteric artery (SMA), and in rare cases where this is not an option, the celiac and, lastly, the inferior mesenteric artery (IMA) can be targeted. Evidence from multiple sources supports an endovascular-first approach for these patients. Endovascular approach with stents and angioplasty leads to better short-term outcomes but a higher rate of recurrent symptoms requiring reintervention [14]. However, in some patients, the anatomy of the mesenteric vessels does not allow for this approach, and a traditional open operation may be needed. The preferred approach will depend on the anatomy and the patient's condition. The preferred choice for inflow is the supra celiac aorta, as it allows for antegrade flow, and the celiac tends to be free from atherosclerosis, but this requires more extensive dissection and risk associated with aortic cross-clamping. In cases where this is not possible, retrograde bypasses from the infrarenal aorta or the iliac vessels are an option. In terms of conduit, prosthetic grafts have similar patency and outcomes to autologous grafts, but no additional vein harvest is required, and they are more versatile.

In patients with AMI, the patients usually present in worse condition and require expeditious revascularization to preserve as much bowel as possible. Recent guidelines from the World Society of Emergency Surgery recommend endovascular revascularization procedures as the primary option in cases of arterial occlusion when sufficient expertise is available. (Strong recommendation based on low-quality evidence 1C) [15]. If unable to use endovascular techniques, a hybrid approach during exploratory laparotomy with a retrograde open mesenteric stenting provides revascularization faster than a bypass with similar patency and outcomes. But if a bypass is required, it is essential to take into consideration that if there is bowel necrosis or perforation with contamination, there is a higher risk of infection when a prosthetic conduit is used. Consideration should be made of using a saphenous vein or other venous conduits for this purpose.

Carotid Disease

The use of the saphenous vein for carotid disease is rare, and it is mainly reserved for situations where there is a need to replace the internal carotid artery, as seen in cases of infection after previous carotid intervention. The incidence of patch infection is 0.25–0.5% of all carotid endarterectomies; a slightly higher incidence is reported when prosthetic patches are used [16, 17]. Also, infections have been reported on carotid stents within radiated fields with cutaneous fistula formation. Patients can present with acute symptoms like expanding hematoma or pseudoaneurysm to chronic presentations like an abscess or a draining sinus. By far, the most common bacteria involved are S. aureus and S. epidermidis [18]. Because of how rare these infections are, there is no hard evidence on how to treat them. However, the consensus is to treat them similarly to infections in other fields with antibiotics, debridement, and reconstruction with autogenous conduit, avoiding prosthetics when possible. To date, most favor using an autologous vein as the conduit in carotid artery reconstruction, [18] although reconstruction with the superficial femoral artery has been described as an option [19]. When using vein conduits, we favor greater saphenous veins with >4 mm diameter and appropriate thickness to decrease the risk of subsequent CVA and aneurysmal degeneration [20].

Superficial Venous Insufficiency with Concomitant Deep Reflux

Deep venous pathology, including reflux and obstruction, can affect outcomes of saphenous vein treatments; therefore, according to the most recent SVS/AVF guidelines, evaluation of the deep venous system is recommended in symptomatic patients with C2 disease and above [1].

In a large retrospective trial by Brow et al., 4881 patients who underwent endovenous ablation were identified on the Vascular Quality Initiative database; 46.2% had combined superficial and deep reflux. After long-term follow-up, all patients had improvement in symptoms, and the combined reflux patients had more significant improvement in Venous Clinical Severity Scores (VCSS) and similar DVT rates but a higher risk of overall complications, including paresthesia, skin pigmentation, superficial phlebitis, wound infection, and proximal thrombus extension [21]. Other investigators also have similar improvements in venous ulcer healing rates after endovenous ablation in patients with and without concomitant deep vein reflux, highlighting the importance of superficial reflux treatment regardless of the presence of deep reflux [22]. Interestingly, in this study, the resolution of segmental deep vein reflux after superficial vein surgery was also noted in 49% of patients. Patients with significant femoral or popliteal reflux velocity of >10 cm/s or severe deep venous reflux (considered as three-segment incompetence in the common femoral, femoral, and popliteal veins) have a higher risk of persistent symptoms and recanalization [4, 23].

Superficial Venous Insufficiency with Concomitant Deep Venous Obstruction

- There is a paucity of significant data regarding saphenous vein interruption with concomitant proximal obstruction, secondary to a general apprehension from most surgeons of treating the superficial veins in these patients due to the theoretical risk of worsening venous flow [1]. When the femoral vein is obstructed, the profunda femoral venous system takes a more dominant role in collateralization. In contrast, iliac vein collateralization is sparser and functionally poorer, depending on neovascularization over time. Due to this, some support first correcting the proximal venous outflow obstruction. Regardless, the GSV has little collateral role in femoral or iliac vein occlusions, and therefore, it is safe to ablate. Although the level of evidence is weak, Raju et al. showed in two small series that patients with different degrees of deep vein obstruction, mostly post-thrombotic syndrome, have good outcomes following saphenous ablation, with improvement in reflux without worsening obstruction parameters [24, 25]. In patients with previous DVT, it is also safe to perform endovenous ablations, as suggested by Puggione et al. in their review of 29 patients without increased incidence of thrombotic complications following radiofrequency ablation (RFA) of the GSV [26].

Klippel-Trenaunay Syndrome (KTS)

KTS is a congenital venous malformation characterized by the classic triad of limb hypertrophy, varicose veins, and port wine stain [27]. They can present with complications like venous ulcers, thrombophlebitis, DVT, PE, and bleeding varicosities [28]. Nonoperative medical management is the preferred modality to treat KTS, but in patients who fail to respond, surgical management is accepted [29]. Open surgical treatment has been described successfully with a good clinical response, with the understanding that one-fourth of patients will require secondary procedures [30]. Minimally invasive procedures are the most current approach to KTS, including angioplasty and stenting of the deep venous system, superficial endovenous ablation, sclerotherapy, and phlebectomy when needed [28, 29].

Before treating truncal reflux in these patients, the patency of the deep system should be documented, particularly in those with a persistent lateral marginal or sciatic vein. This is an embryonic remanent present in patients with KTS and could be the main outflow for the lower extremity. Removal of this pathway can lead to worsening symptoms. When choosing an intervention, preference should be given to sclerotherapy or embolization, particularly for superficial veins, to avoid palpable cords or thermal skin injuries. This is also true for the sciatic vein due to the proximity to the nerve [31, 32].

GSV Preserving Interventions

In the most recent guidelines for the management of varicose veins, two procedures are described and recommended when attempting to preserve the greater saphenous vein in early stage patients with symptomatic varicose veins: the ASVAL and CHIVA techniques [1]. Both approaches require a trained surgeon who is familiar with the procedure and has good ultrasound skills.

Ambulatory Selective Variceal Ablation Under Local Anesthesia (ASVAL)

These operations are based on the "ascending theory," suggesting that the venous disease process starts in the tributaries and distal truncal veins and then progresses into the junction and deep system [33]. In this procedure, the GSV tributaries are carefully mapped to the truncal GSV using ultrasound and removed under local anesthesia using a microphlebectomy technique. A recent randomized trial, the SAPTAP trial, compared this technique against traditional treatment with phlebectomy and concomitant ablation, showing similar improvement of symptoms and anatomical results in the short term, but 25% of patients will have a recurrence of symptoms in 9 months' follow-up, requiring ablation of the truncal vein [34]. Certainly, the other way to interpret this is that the truncal vein was preserved in 75% of these patients. Other studies have also shown improvement in the volume of superficial and deep reflux following this procedure [35].

Conservative and Hemodynamic Ambulatory Treatment of Venous Insufficiency (CHIVA)

CHIVA is the French acronym for "Cure conservatrice et Hemodynamique de l'Insuffisance Veineuse en Ambulatoire." This procedure was designed to improve hemodynamic insufficiency while avoiding the removal of tributaries. The goal is to correct abnormal hemodynamic pathways identified on a very detailed ultrasound mapping. This technique requires identifying the venous-venous shunts, or where the reflux starts (commonly referred to as venous escape points), and ligating them under local anesthesia without removing the tributaries. It is crucial to identify the reentry points (i.e., perforators), as this will lead to a stagnant column of blood in the vein that could potentially lead to thrombosis of the saphenous vein [36]. This is why the ultrasound examination needs to be extremely nuanced to identify all these specifics preoperatively. There have been randomized trials that show CHIVA has less recurrence compared to GSV stripping [37]. On a Cochrane review, with a low to very low level of certainty, CHIVA showed similar outcomes when compared to stripping or endovenous thermal ablation of the GSV but may result in more bruising when compared to RFA. It should be noted that these conclusions are based on a small number of trials with fewer events, and more randomized clinical trials may be needed [38].

Conclusion

There is clear evidence of the benefit of surgical treatment of the saphenous vein in patients with symptomatic venous insufficiency. Still, it is important to understand the nuance and anatomic complexity of venous reflux when deciding our treatment approach and the concomitant finding of deep venous involvement. We also need to consider the preservation of saphenous veins in patients at higher risk of peripheral or coronary artery disease who may need it as a conduit for revascularization.

Summary

There is strong evidence supporting the advantages of treating the saphenous vein in patients experiencing symptomatic superficial venous insufficiency. However, the saphenous vein is not just a potential source of pathology; it also holds significant value as a potential graft for future vascular surgeries. It is crucial to recognize the nuances and anatomical complexities of venous reflux when determining the appropriate treatment strategy. Coronary Artery Bypass Graft (CABG), Peripheral Artery Disease (PAD), and concurrent deep venous pathology are among other conditions that warrant special consideration. Preservation of the saphenous vein should not be done at the expense of sacrificing quality of life, but ablation must consider the challenges in the management of high-risk patients.

References

1. Gloviczki P, et al. The 2023 Society for Vascular Surgery, American Venous Forum, and American Vein and Lymphatic Society clinical practice guidelines for the management of varicose veins of the lower extremities. Part II: Endorsed by the Society of Interventional Radiology and the Society for Vascular Medicine. J Vasc Surg Venous Lymphat Disord. 2024;12(1):101670.
2. Natour AK, Kabbani L. Femoral-popliteal bypass graft. In: Hans SS, Weaver MR, Nypaver TJ, editors. Primary and repeat arterial reconstructions. Cham: Springer; 2023. https://doi.org/10.1007/978-3-031-13897-3_32.
3. Obiweluozor FO, Emechebe GA, Kim DW, et al. Considerations in the development of small-diameter vascular graft as an alternative for bypass and reconstructive surgeries: a review. Cardiovasc Eng Tech. 2020;11:495–521. https://doi.org/10.1007/s13239-020-00482-y.
4. Akca F, Lam KY, Verberkmoes N, de Lathauwer I, Soliman-Hamad M, van Straten B. Predictive value of great saphenous vein mapping prior to endoscopic harvesting in coronary artery bypass surgery. Interact CardioVascular Thorac Surg. 31(1):16–9. https://doi.org/10.1093/icvts/ivaa063.
5. Farber A, et al. Surgery or endovascular therapy for chronic limb-threatening ischemia. N Engl J Med. 2022;387(25):2305–16.
6. Synovec JD, Walton ZJ, Leddy LR, Suleiman LI, Gross CE. Notable racial and ethnic disparities persist in lower extremity amputations for critical limb ischemia and infection. J Am Acad Orthop Surg. 2020;28(21):885–92. https://doi.org/10.5435/JAAOS-D-19-00630.
7. Butala NM, Chandra V, Beckman JA, Parikh SA, Lookstein R, Misra S, Secemsky EA. Contextualizing the BEST-CLI trial results in clinical practice. J Soc Cardiovasc Angiogr Interv. 2023;2(4):101036. https://doi.org/10.1016/j.jscai.2023.101036.
8. Gornik HL, Aronow HD, Goodney PP, Arya S, Brewster LP, Byrd L, Chandra V, Drachman DE, Eaves JM, Ehrman JK, Evans JN, Getchius TSD, Gutiérrez JA, Hawkins BM, Hess CN, Ho KJ, Jones WS, Kim ESH, Kinlay S, Kirksey L, Kohlman-Trigoboff D, Long CA, Pollak AW, Sabri SS, Sadwin LB, Secemsky EA, Serhal M, Shishehbor MH, Treat-Jacobson D, Wilkins LR. 2024 ACC/AHA/AACVPR/APMA/ABC/SCAI/SVM/SVN/SVS/SIR/VESS guideline for the management of lower extremity peripheral artery disease: a report of the American College of Cardiology/American Heart Association Joint Committee on Clinical Practice Guidelines. Circulation. 2024;149(24):e1313–410.
9. Nastasi DR, Moxon JV, Norman R, Trollope AF, Rowbotham S, Quigley F, Jenkins J, Golledge J. The cost-effectiveness of intensive low-density

lipoprotein cholesterol lowering in people with peripheral artery disease. J Vasc Surg. 2021;73(4):1396–1403.e3.
10. Bonaca MP, Nault P, Giugliano RP, Keech AC, Pineda AL, Kanevsky E, Kuder J, Murphy SA, Jukema JW, Lewis BS, Tokgozoglu L, Somaratne R, Sever PS, Pedersen TR, Sabatine MS. Low-density lipoprotein cholesterol lowering with evolocumab and outcomes in patients with peripheral artery disease: insights from the FOURIER Trial (Further cardiovascular outcomes research with PCSK9 inhibition in subjects with elevated risk). Circulation. 2018;137(4):338–50.
11. Bonaca MP, Bauersachs RM, Anand SS, Debus ES, Nehler MR, Patel MR, Fanelli F, Capell WH, Diao L, Jaeger N, Hess CN, Pap AF, Kittelson JM, Gudz I, Mátyás L, Krievins DK, Diaz R, Brodmann M, Muehlhofer E, Haskell LP, Berkowitz SD, Hiatt WR. Rivaroxaban in peripheral artery disease after revascularization. N Engl J Med. 2020;382(21):1994–2004.
12. Serruys PW, et al. Percutaneous coronary intervention versus coronary-artery bypass grafting for severe coronary artery disease. N Engl J Med. 2009;360(10):961–72.
13. Farkouh ME, et al. Strategies for multivessel revascularization in patients with diabetes. N Engl J Med. 2012;367(25):2375–84.
14. Huber TS, et al. Chronic mesenteric ischemia: clinical practice guidelines from the Society for Vascular Surgery. J Vasc Surg. 2021;73(1S):87S–115S.
15. Bala M, et al. Acute mesenteric ischemia: updated guidelines of the World Society of Emergency Surgery. World J Emerg Surg. 2022;17(1):54.
16. Hayes PD, et al. Randomized trial of vein versus Dacron patching during carotid endarterectomy: influence of patch type on postoperative embolization. J Vasc Surg. 2001;33(5):994–1000.
17. Naylor AR, et al. Prosthetic patch infection after carotid endarterectomy. Eur J Vasc Endovasc Surg. 2002;23(1):11–6.
18. Knight BC, Tait WF. Dacron patch infection following carotid endarterectomy: a systematic review of the literature. Eur J Vasc Endovasc Surg. 2009;37(2):140–8.
19. Naughton PA, et al. Carotid artery reconstruction for infected carotid patches. Eur J Vasc Endovasc Surg. 2010;40(4):492–8.
20. Guerra A, et al. Ipsilateral carotid bypass outcomes in hostile neck anatomy. J Vasc Surg. 2021;74(6):1929–36.
21. Brown CS, et al. Effect of concomitant deep venous reflux on truncal endovenous ablation outcomes in the Vascular Quality Initiative. J Vasc Surg Venous Lymphat Disord. 2021;9(2):361–368 e3.
22. Adam DJ, et al. Role of superficial venous surgery in patients with combined superficial and segmental deep venous reflux. Eur J Vasc Endovasc Surg. 2003;25(5):469–72.
23. Meissner MH, Natiello C, Nicholls SC. Performance characteristics of the venous clinical severity score. J Vasc Surg. 2002;36(5):889–95.

24. Raju S, et al. Saphenectomy in the presence of chronic venous obstruction. Surgery. 1998;123(6):637–44.
25. Lawton JS, Tamis-Holland JE, Bangalore S, Bates ER, Beckie TM, Mischoff JM, et al. ACC/AHA/SCAI guideline for coronary artery revascularization, a report of the American College of Cardiology/American Heart Association Joint Committee on clinical practice guidelines. J Am Coll Cardiol. 2021;2022:79.
26. Puggioni A, et al. The safety of radiofrequency ablation of the great saphenous vein in patients with previous venous thrombosis. J Vasc Surg. 2009;49(5):1248–55.
27. Sermsathanasawadi N, et al. Endovenous radiofrequency thermal ablation and ultrasound-guided foam sclerotherapy in treatment of klippel-trenaunay syndrome. Ann Vasc Dis. 2014;7(1):52–5.
28. Saleem T, Luke C, Raju S. Options in the treatment of superficial and deep venous disease in patients with Klippel-Trenaunay syndrome. J Vasc Surg Venous Lymphat Disord. 2022;10(6):1343–1351 e3.
29. Wang SK, et al. Diagnosis and management of the venous malformations of Klippel-Trenaunay syndrome. J Vasc Surg Venous Lymphat Disord. 2017;5(4):587–95.
30. Malgor RD, et al. Surgical treatment of varicose veins and venous malformations in Klippel-Trenaunay syndrome. Phlebology. 2016;31(3):209–15.
31. Group KW. Clinical practice guidelines for Klippel Trenaunay Syndrome. Boston Children Hospital; 2016.
32. Frasier K, et al. Endovascular radiofrequency ablation: a novel treatment of venous insufficiency in Klippel-Trenaunay patients. J Vasc Surg. 2008;47(6):1339–45.
33. Onida S, Davies AH. CHIVA, ASVAL and related techniques – concepts and evidence. Phlebology. 2015;30(2 Suppl):42–5.
34. Scheerders ERY, et al. A randomized clinical trial of isolated ambulatory phlebectomy versus saphenous thermal ablation with concomitant phlebectomy (SAPTAP Trial). Br J Surg. 2023;110(3):333–42.
35. Pittaluga P, et al. The effect of isolated phlebectomy on reflux and diameter of the great saphenous vein: a prospective study. Eur J Vasc Endovasc Surg. 2010;40(1):122–8.
36. Faccini FP, Ermini S, Franceschi C. CHIVA to treat saphenous vein insufficiency in chronic venous disease: characteristics and results. J Vasc Bras. 2019;18:e20180099.
37. Carandina S, et al. Varicose vein stripping vs haemodynamic correction (CHIVA): a long term randomised trial. Eur J Vasc Endovasc Surg. 2008;35(2):230–7.
38. Bellmunt-Montoya S, et al. CHIVA method for the treatment of chronic venous insufficiency. Cochrane Database Syst Rev. 2021;9(9):CD009648.

6 Vascular Medicine for the Venous Specialist

M. Ihsan Kaadan and Carlos Echevarria

A 72-year-old male patient with a past medical history of CAD, DM, HTN, and HLD underwent a coronary angiography procedure. Several days later, the patient developed severe pain in the toes. Upon further investigation, the underlying cause was found to be cholesterol emboli that had been dislodged during the procedure, leading to downstream blockage and reduced blood flow.

Anatomy of the Disease: Blue Toe Syndrome

Blue toe syndrome (BTS) can have several underlying causes that range from benign to life-threatening conditions. First reported in the literature in 1976 by Komody et al., it described 31 cases

M. I. Kaadan
Division of Cardiology, Department of Medicine, Rush University Medical Center, Chicago, IL, USA
e-mail: M.ihsan_kaadan@rush.edu

C. Echevarria (✉)
Division of Vascular and Endovascular Surgery, Department of Surgery, Massachusetts General Hospital/Harvard Venous & Lymphatic Medicine Alumni, Boston, MA, USA

Division of Vascular Medicine and Endovenous Interventions, Veins & Vascular Centers of Excellence, Phoenix, AZ, USA
e-mail: carlos.echevarria@vascular.md

C. Echevarria et al. (eds.), *The Massachusetts General Hospital Protocols and Procedures for Venous Disease*,
https://doi.org/10.1007/978-3-032-05708-2_6

caused by multiple etiologies, many from proximal lesions in the arterial tree that serve as probable sources of emboli, causing microembolization to the digital arteries. However, not all cases were caused by proximal lesions in the arterial tree, which calls for an analysis of the differential diagnosis [1].

Differential Diagnosis

BTS may indicate impaired blood flow or oxygenation to the affected area. In order to classify and better understand alternative etiologies, we have organized them into three different categories: arterial inflow disease, venous outflow disease, and inherited blood conditions [2] (see Fig. 6.1).

Arterial Inflow Disease

Peripheral Vascular Disease

Peripheral Arterial Disease (PAD): When a stenosis or occlusion of the peripheral arteries reaches a critical point, it could lead to impaired blood flow to the extremities. Patients with PAD may be asymptomatic, although this may be due to lack of demand, as it frequently happens in the elderly. Some patients, when exerted, may develop intermittent claudication. More advanced disease may present with rest pain or non-healing ulcers, typically located on the toes or feet, with trophic changes on the lower limb, including hair loss, nail dystrophy, and diminished or absent peripheral pulses. Some patients may present with leg pain only when lying in bed. Such complaints may represent atypical symptoms of advanced disease due to poor perfusion when elevating the legs and may require further evaluation.

Thrombosis: Although arterial thrombosis is not as common as venous thromboembolism, it can have serious consequences, leading to acutely reduced blood flow to the extremities and blue toes due to tissue hypoxia. Acute arterial thrombosis could be driven by different conditions, including antiphospholipid syndrome, disseminated intravascular coagulation, COVID thrombosis, and warfarin-induced skin necrosis.

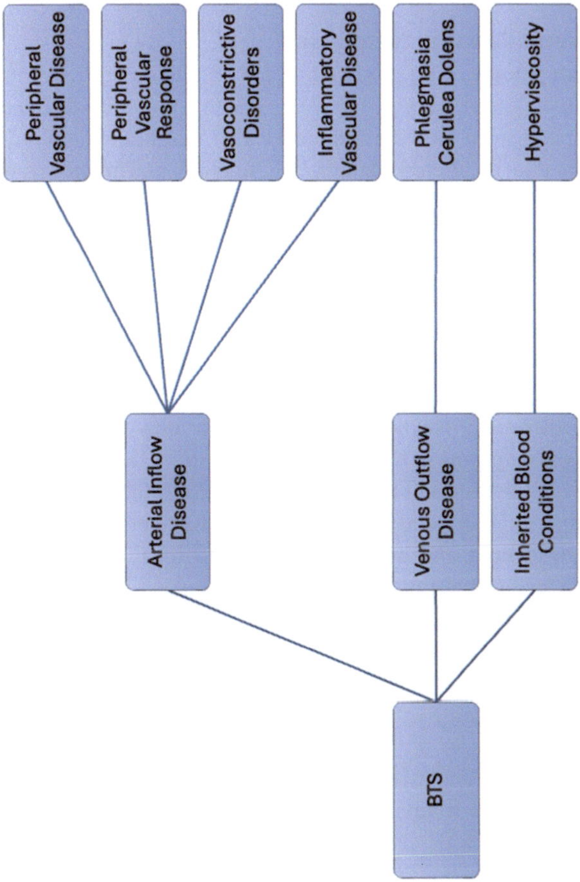

Fig. 6.1 Blue toe syndrome classification based on etiology

Embolism: Thrombi can break off and travel to peripheral arteries, blocking blood flow to the toes and causing a blue discoloration. This can occur after vascular procedures as an iatrogenic complication or due to other underlying conditions such as cardiac emboli or endocarditis.

Peripheral Vascular Response

Sepsis or Shock: The most significant finding on these events is widespread vasodilation, decreasing systemic vascular resistance and hypotension. However, there is also microcirculatory dysfunction due to altered endothelial function and microthrombi formation, affecting blood flow at the capillary level.

Vasoconstrictive Disorders

Medication-Induced Ischemia: Investigate potential side effects of warfarin, beta-blockers, and ergot derivatives, as well as other drugs, including cocaine and amphetamines.

Acrosyndromes: Raynaud's phenomenon may occur due to blood vessel spasms in response to cold or stress, leading to color changes in the toes and fingers, whereas pernio (chilblains) is an inflammatory skin condition that occurs in response to repeated exposure to cold and humidity, leading to localized erythema, swelling, and sometimes ulceration. Acrocyanosis is another condition affecting the extremities that can be confused with Raynaud's phenomenon and pernio. It is characterized by persistent, painless cyanosis of the hands and feet, typically without associated ischemic symptoms or progression to ulcers (Fig. 6.2.

Inflammatory Vascular Disease

Vasculitis: It is a heterogeneous group of disorders that can lead to vessel wall damage, luminal narrowing, occlusion, aneurysm formation, and rupture. Vasculitis can affect vessels of any size, type, and location and can be primary or secondary to other conditions. The underlying mechanism involves immune-mediated injury to the vessel wall caused by genetic predisposition, environmental triggers, and immune system

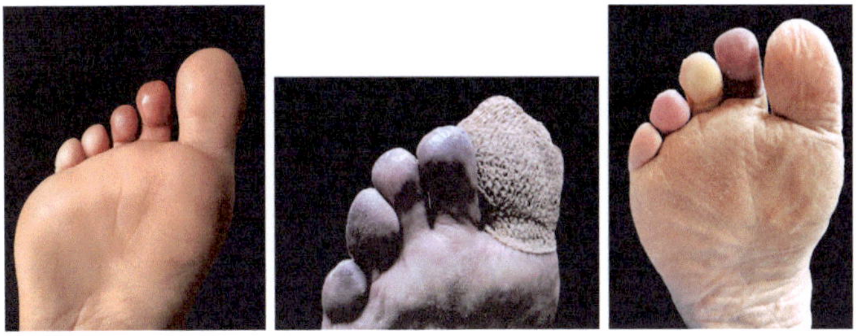

Fig. 6.2 Pernio (left): notice the erythema that could lead to ulcerative lesions on the tips of the toes. Acrocyanosis (middle): notice vasoconstriction that eventually evolves into bluish discoloration; usually benign. Raynaud (right): when exposed to cold, an extreme reactive vasoconstriction will ensue. Notice the initial pale reaction (3rd toe) evolving into bluish discoloration (2nd toe) and erythema (4th toe) upon blood flow return

dysregulation (Fig. 6.3). A classic etiology for BTS is Buerger's disease. Also called thromboangiitis obliterans, it is often associated with heavy smoking, causing inflammation and clotting of peripheral toe blood vessels (Buerger's disease may also be present in the fingers).

Calcific vasculopathy, or "calciphylaxis," Refers to the abnormal buildup of calcium deposits in the vessel walls, commonly as a complication or associated with an inflammatory response. This can lead to reduced blood flow to the skin and soft tissue necrosis and gangrene. It most commonly affects patients with end-stage renal disease or those undergoing long-term dialysis. This condition is also associated with autoimmune connective tissue disease.

Venous Outflow Disease

DVT and phlegmasia cerulea dolens can lead to complications affecting blood flow to the toes due to extensive venous thrombosis. The blockage causes severe venous hypertension, leading to severe swelling and tissue edema. This can compromise nearby arterial flow, leading to ischemia and potential gangrene.

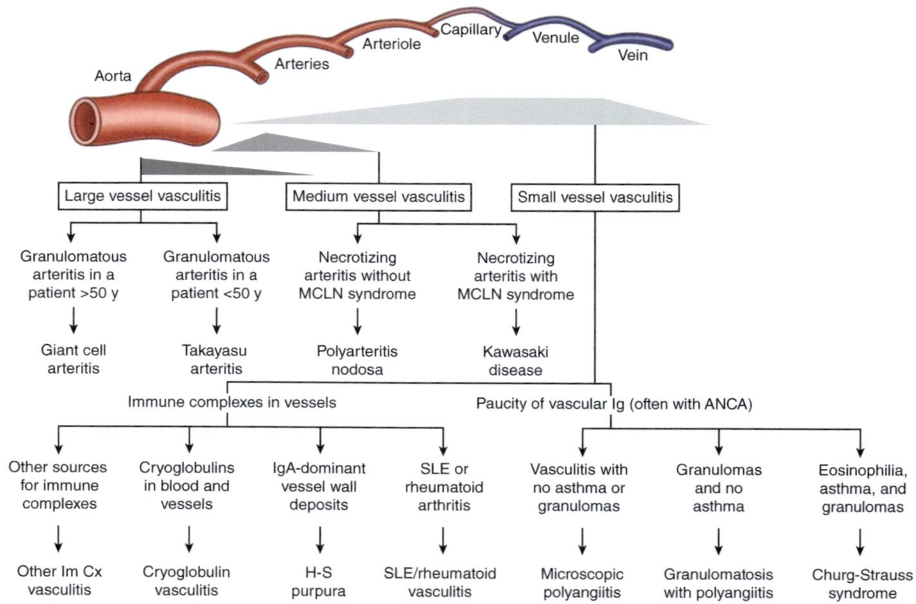

Fig. 6.3 Illustration showing the most common vasculitides based on the size of the artery or vein affected. MCLN, mucocutaneous lymph node syndrome; ANCA, antineutrophil cytoplasmic antibody; Im Cx, immune complex; H-S purpura, Henoch-Schönlein purpura; SLE, systemic lupus erythematosus. (Modified from Ref. [3])

Blood Disorders

Hyperviscosity is the main causative event that leads to impaired blood flow, promoting thrombosis and embolism of the small arteries in the toes, leading to the blue discoloration characteristic of blue toe syndrome. This can be seen in conditions like myeloproliferative disorders, polycythemia vera, essential thrombocythemia, cryoglobulinemia, and cold agglutinins.

Diagnostic and Management

Auxilliary Testing/Imaging Studies

Diagnosis typically involves carefully reviewing the patient's medical history and performing a complete physical examination. This comprehensive approach helps identify the root cause of symptoms and guides further decisions in conducting relevant tests.

History

- Collect information about the onset and progression of symptoms, including when the toes became blue or discolored—the relationship of the symptom's onset to weather changes.
- Inquire about other symptoms such as pain, tingling, numbness, or weakness in the affected area.
- Gather details about past medical history, including existing vascular conditions, diabetes, hypertension, hyperlipidemia, smoking, or other risk factors.
- Carefully review the patient's medication list.
- Ask about recent surgeries, particularly vascular or cardiac procedures, which could be related to thromboembolic events.
- Inquire about any family history of aneurysms, genetic disease, thrombotic or blood disorders.

Physical Examination

1. **Distribution of Affected Toes**
   - **Single or Few Toes Affected**: More typical of embolic events (e.g., from atherosclerotic plaque or cardiac sources).
   - **Symmetrical Involvement of Multiple Toes**: Suggests a systemic condition like Raynaud's phenomenon or acrocyanosis.
   - **Tip-Sparing Discoloration**: Inquire about trauma. Differentiate from Achenbach syndrome, an intermittent spontaneous tip-sparing ecchymosis-like conditions, suspected to be related to increased vascular fragility.
2. **Temperature and Moisture**
   - **Cold, Clammy Skin**: Suggests ongoing ischemia, common in acrocyanosis, frostbite, and severe Raynaud's. Identify symmetric peripheral pulses.
   - **Warm Skin with Color Changes**: More consistent with vasculitis or an inflammatory process.
3. **Color Changes**
   - **Blue/Purplish Discoloration**: Sudden onset of blue or purple color in one or more toes is characteristic of BTS. Determine acuity and time to resolution for potential differential diagnoses. Raised, red, or purple lesions can suggest pernio (chilblains), mainly if they occur after exposure to cold and damp conditions.
   - **Triphasic Color Changes (White-Blue-Red)**: This pattern is indicative of Raynaud's phenomenon, especially when triggered by cold or stress. It usually involves bilateral, symmetrical episodes.
   - **Non-blanching Purpura**: Suggests vasculitis or other causes of small vessel inflammation and occlusion.
4. **Skin Integrity**
   - **Intact Skin with Cyanosis**: More indicative of acrocyanosis, with persistent cyanosis without ulceration or significant pain.

- **Skin Breakdown and Ulcers:** Suggest more severe ischemia and possible underlying PAD or severe microembolization.
- **Necrosis and Dry Gangrene**: Typically presents as black, mummified tissue and is associated with severe, chronic ischemia, often due to atherosclerosis or thromboangiitis obliterans (Buerger's disease).

5. **Nail Changes**
   - **Dystrophic Nails**: Long-term ischemia can cause nail dystrophy, indicating chronic conditions such as PAD or repeated episodes of Raynaud's.
   - **Splinter Hemorrhages:** Can be seen in subacute bacterial endocarditis, which might lead to embolic events causing BTS.

Diagnostic Tests

Auxiliary blood tests can provide critical information in the differential diagnosis of BTS by identifying underlying systemic conditions, detecting markers of inflammation, assessing coagulation status, and revealing specific hematologic disorders. Here is how various blood tests can aid in the differential diagnosis:

1. **Complete Blood Count (CBC)**
   - **Polycythemia**: Elevated red blood cell count and hemoglobin/hematocrit levels suggest polycythemia vera, which increases blood viscosity and the risk of thrombosis.
   - **Leukocytosis**: Elevated white blood cell count can indicate infection or inflammatory conditions such as vasculitis.
   - **Thrombocytosis**: A high platelet count suggests essential thrombocythemia, another condition associated with increased thrombotic risk.
   - **Anemia**: This can be associated with chronic diseases or hemolytic processes, which might contribute to ischemic symptoms.

2. **Coagulation Profile**
   - **Prothrombin Time (PT) and Activated Partial Thromboplastin Time (aPTT)**: Assess for abnormalities in the coagulation cascade, which can indicate bleeding or thrombotic disorders.
   - **D-Dimer**: Elevated levels suggest recent or ongoing thrombosis, indicating a hypercoagulable state or recent embolic events. Note that D-dimer is a non-specific biomarker that may be present in other proinflammatory conditions.
3. **Inflammatory Markers**
   - **Erythrocyte Sedimentation Rate (ESR) and C-Reactive Protein (CRP)**: Elevated levels are nonspecific markers of inflammation and can indicate vasculitis, infection, or other inflammatory conditions.
4. **Blood Glucose and Glycated Hemoglobin (HbA1c)**
   - **Diabetes Mellitus**: Elevated levels indicate poor glucose control, which is a risk factor for peripheral artery disease (PAD) and microvascular complications that can present as blue toe syndrome.
5. **Renal Function Tests**
   - **Creatinine and Blood Urea Nitrogen (BUN)**: Elevated levels can indicate chronic kidney disease, which is associated with increased cardiovascular risk and can contribute to atheroembolism.
6. **Lipid Profile**
   - **Cholesterol and Triglycerides**: High levels suggest hyperlipidemia, a significant risk factor for atherosclerosis and subsequent embolic events.
7. **Urinalysis**
   - **Urinalysis**: Look for eosinophil cells when atheroemboli is in the differential diagnosis. The presence of cholesterol crystals in the microvasculature induces the release of pro-inflammatory cytokines and chemokines, which recruit eosinophils to the affected tissues, including the kidneys.
8. **Serum Protein Electrophoresis (SPEP) and Immunofixation**

- **Monoclonal Proteins**: Detection of monoclonal gammopathy suggests multiple myeloma or Waldenström's macroglobulinemia, both of which can lead to hyperviscosity and increase the risk of small vessel occlusion.

9. **Autoimmune and Vasculitis Screening**
   - **Antinuclear Antibodies (ANA)**: Positive ANA suggests an underlying autoimmune condition, such as systemic lupus erythematosus (SLE), which can cause vasculitis.
   - **Anti-neutrophil Cytoplasmic Antibodies (ANCA)**: Positive ANCA indicates ANCA-associated vasculitis, which can cause small vessel occlusion and ischemia.
   - **Rheumatoid Factor (RF) and Anti-cyclic Citrullinated Peptide (Anti-CCP) Antibodies**: Elevated levels suggest rheumatoid arthritis, which can be associated with vasculitis.
10. **Specific Hematologic Tests**
    - **JAK2 Mutation Analysis**: Positive in polycythemia vera and essential thrombocythemia, supporting a diagnosis of myeloproliferative disorders.
    - **Cryoglobulins**: Cryoglobulins indicate cryoglobulinemia, which can lead to vasculitis and small vessel occlusion.
    - **Serum Viscosity**: Direct measurement can confirm hyperviscosity syndromes such as Waldenström's macroglobulinemia or multiple myeloma.
11. **Additional Tests and Imaging**
    - **Ankle-Brachial Index (ABI):** The highest systolic blood pressure at the ankle (dorsalis pedis vs. posterior tibialis) divided by the highest systolic pressure of the left and right arm constitutes the ABI. An ABI of ≤0.90 is confirmatory of PAD. If ABI>0.90 but clinical suspicion of PAD remains high, consider postexercise ABI. A postexercise ankle pressure decrease of >30 mmHg or a postexercise ABI decrease of >20% is diagnostic for PAD. Consider other noninvasive tests for further assessment.
    - **Electrocardiogram (ECG) and Cardiac Monitoring**: To rule out cardiac arrhythmias such as atrial fibrillation.

- **Echocardiogram**: To assess cardiac function and other related embolic sources such as endocarditis.
- **Doppler Ultrasound**: To assess blood flow, location, and degree of stenosis, occlusion, or thrombosis if suspecting DVT.
- **Computed Tomography, Magnetic Resonance, Angiogram/Venogram**: Contrast studies used for aneurysm characterization, structural issues, atherosclerotic plaques as a source of emboli, and stenosis.
- **Skin Biopsy**: Although rarely used, it may help rule out conditions such as calciphylaxis or vasculitis.

Management

Medical Management

Endovascular/Surgical Interventions

- CAPRIE (1996): Clopidogrel vs. aspirin in CV disease
- INTERHEART (2004) Modifiable risk factors
- TNT (2005): Atorvastatin in stable CAD
- CHARISMA (2006): Aspirin/clopidogrel vs. aspirin for CV prevention
- JUPITER (2008): Rosuvastatin for primary CV prevention
- VOYAGER-PAD (2020): Rivaroxaban 2.5 mg BID in PAD

Managing blue toes depends on the underlying cause and severity of symptoms. Since blue toes often indicate compromised blood flow, the management approach requires immediate medical evaluation and stabilization. Once the chances of further complications have been minimized, management should be tailored to address the root cause. A detailed discussion of the care of all potential etiologies of blue toe syndrome is outside of the scope of this chapter, but we will focus our attention on PAD management.

Peripheral Arterial Disease (PAD)

Lifestyle changes, such as smoking cessation, diet, and exercise, remain the cornerstone of PAD management. However, advancements in pharmacological therapies have dramatically improved outcomes.

Until 1996, the cornerstone of PAD pharmacological management was defined by a hundred-year-old drug: aspirin. Although aspirin has remained relevant to this date, the CAPRIE study identified clopidogrel as an alternative treatment, showing better efficacy for preventing MACE with similar bleeding rates compared to aspirin [4]. Since then, other antiplatelets, such as ticagrelor, have been tested, showing somewhat similar efficacy outcomes to clopidogrel but with higher rates of adverse events [5]. Most recently, the VOYAGER-PAD trial demonstrated superior outcomes when rivaroxaban 2.5 mg BID was added to antiplatelet therapy, reducing the risk of MACE and MALE [6]. This regimen has now been ratified as first-line therapy for PAD in the most recent guidelines.

The TNT and JUPITER studies established statins as a key component in the treatment regimen, showing a reduction in the incidence of MALE, cardiovascular, and all-cause mortality in patients with PAD [7].

Blood pressure management is recommended to reduce rates of cardiovascular disease and associated mortality for patients with PAD (current goals of <130/80 mmHg). ACE inhibitors are the agent of choice, especially for those with a history of diabetes mellitus [8]. Special consideration to calcium channel blockers as first-line therapy for African Americans [9, 10].

Monitored exercise program is recommended for all patients unless contraindicated. Cilostazol can be considered for symptoms control if not contraindicated (avoid using it in heart failure).

In severe cases, despite optimized medical therapy, revascularization is indicated in patients with acute limb ischemia (ALI) and a salvageable limb to prevent irreversible tissue damage and major amputation.

The management of blue toes can vary significantly based on the underlying cause, so a comprehensive evaluation is crucial to determine the most appropriate treatment plan.

Surveillance

Regular Check-Ups: Follow-up to monitor progress and side effects such as active bleeding and adjust treatments as needed, especially when anticoagulation has been added to the treatment regimen.

Complications and Management

Smoking has been associated with an increased risk of PAD, even as a secondhand smoker (RR 1.67) or after cessation (although this correlation diminishes beyond 10 years after quitting). Interestingly, the anatomic distribution of the disease tends to be more axial, while patients with diabetes have a more distal disease distribution. Patients with PAD and uncontrolled diabetes have a fivefold increased risk of amputation when compared to non-diabetic PAD patients. Clearly, atherosclerotic disease is not limited to the lower limbs. Patients with PAD have at least an additional threefold risk of cardiovascular disease or cerebrovascular events [11, 12].

Key Point Synopsis

The case presented at the beginning of this chapter underscores the importance of recognizing iatrogenic causes of blue toe syndrome, especially following vascular or cardiac procedures, but also emphasizes the importance of broad knowledge in the differential diagnoses of blue toe syndrome, as discussed throughout this chapter.

Summary

The pathophysiology of blue toe syndrome has several underlying causes that range from benign to life-threatening conditions. In this chapter, we organized them into three different categories: arterial inflow disease, venous outflow disease, and inherited blood conditions. Proper history and identification of distribution, temperature, skin integrity, and color changes aid in proper diagnosis and specific management. Acuity will help with the differential diagnosis, where conditions such as acrosyndromes will commonly have a sudden onset, while vasculitis will have a more surreptitious presentation. Although many conditions are self-limited, peripheral vascular disease tends to be progressive and warrants aggressive medical management.

References

1. Karmody AM, Powers SR, Monaco VJ, Leather RP. "Blue toe" syndrome: an indication for limb salvage surgery. Arch Surg. 1976;111(11):1263–8. https://doi.org/10.1001/archsurg.1976.01360290097015.
2. Hirschmann JV, Raugi GJ. Blue (or purple) toe syndrome. J Am Acad Dermatol. 2009;60(1):1–20.
3. Jennette JC, Falk FJ. Nosology of primary vasculitis. Curr Opin Rheumatol. 2007;19:10.
4. CAPRIE Steering Committee. A randomized, blinded trial of clopidogrel versus aspirin in patients at risk of ischaemic events (CAPRIE). Lancet. 1996;348:1329–39.
5. Hiatt WR, Fowkes FG, Heizer G, et al. Ticagrelor versus clopidogrel in symptomatic peripheral artery disease. N Engl J Med. 2017;376:32–40.
6. Eikelboom JW, Connolly SJ, Bosch J, et al. Rivaroxaban with or without aspirin in stable cardiovascular disease. N Engl J Med. 2017;377:1319–30.
7. Pastori D, Farcomeni A, Milanese A, et al. Statins and major adverse limb events in patients with peripheral artery disease: a systematic review and meta-analysis. Thromb Haemost. 2020;120:866–75.
8. Jude EB, Oyibo SO, Chalmers N, Boulton AJ. Peripheral arterial disease in diabetic and nondiabetic patients: a comparison of severity and outcome. Diabetes Care. 2001;24:1433–7.

9. Sprint Research Group, Wright JT, Williamson JD, et al. A randomized trial of intensive versus standard blood-pressure control. N Engl J Med. 2015;373:2103–16.
10. Mehler PS, Coll JR, Estacio R, et al. Intensive blood pressure control reduces the risk of cardiovascular events in patients with peripheral arterial disease and type 2 diabetes. Circulation. 2003;107:753–6.
11. Newman AB, Siscovick DS, Manolio TA, Polak J, Fried LP, Borhani NO, Wolfson SK. Ankle-arm index as a marker of atherosclerosis in the Cardiovascular Health Study. Cardiovascular Heart Study (CHS) Collaborative Research Group. Circulation. 1993;88:837–45.
12. Joosten MM, Pai JK, Bertoia ML, Rimm EB, Spiegelman D, Mittleman MA, Mukamal KJ. Associations between conventional cardiovascular risk factors and risk of peripheral artery disease in men. JAMA. 2012;308:1660–7. https://doi.org/10.1001/jama.2012.13415.

Part IV

Areas of Special Interest

7 Venous Leg Ulcers

Maureen Walsh McCarthy
and Jeremy Goverman

Venous leg ulcers (VLUs) represent the most common etiology of lower extremity ulcers; as such, they are commonly encountered and treated in our Wound Center. As is the case for all chronic wounds, the healing of a VLU requires a multidisciplinary approach. We regularly see patients for second opinions who may have had non-healing VLUs for months or even years. Rice et al. estimated that 2% of the Medicare population has VLUs (Fig. 7.1).

M. W. McCarthy
Department of Surgery, Massachusetts General Hospital, Lead NP Wound Service, Boston, MA, USA
e-mail: mmccarthy29@mgb.org

J. Goverman (✉)
Department of Surgery, Massachusetts General Hospital, Sumner Redstone Burn Center, Harvard Medical School, Boston, MA, USA
e-mail: Jgoverman@mgb.org

C. Echevarria et al. (eds.), *The Massachusetts General Hospital Protocols and Procedures for Venous Disease*,
https://doi.org/10.1007/978-3-032-05708-2_7

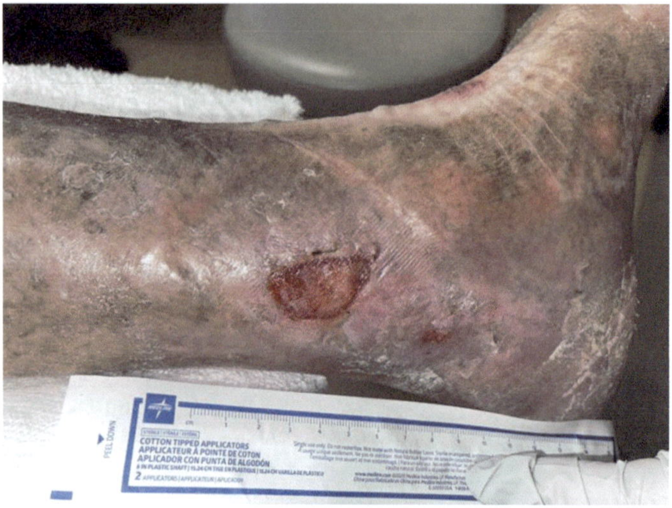

Fig. 7.1 Left medial lower leg venous ulcer

Anatomy of the Disease

The Clinical Picture

Who gets a venous leg ulcer (VLU)? These types of ulcers typically occur in patients with the following risk factors: heredity, venous valve disease, past deep venous thrombosis, history of trauma to the limb, obesity, diabetes, lymphedema, immobility, and advanced age. In the setting of venous insufficiency, Raffetto found that the presence of various inflammatory cells plays a central role in the pathophysiology.

How do we make the diagnosis of a VLU? The physical exam of the patient's lower extremities will likely reveal the stigmata of long-term venous stasis. This includes edema, hemosiderin staining, small varicosities or large tortuous varicose veins, corona phlebectatica, and potentially lipodermatosclerosis, characterized by subcutaneous fibrosis with overlying skin induration. The most common, classic location for a venous ulcer is the medial perimalleolar region. VLUs tend to be shallow with moderate to high volume of exudate and irregular margins. Patients frequently report that the ulcer began after bumping the leg or scratching due to pruritus.

Differential Diagnosis

As with treating any chronic wound/ulcer, the first step in effective treatment is firmly establishing the diagnosis. What is the cause of this ulcer? Is there a problem with the inflow, arterial disease? Is there a problem with outflow, venous disease? Or is it a combination of both? VLUs tend to be associated with low pain levels. Therefore, the presence of high levels of reported pain may indicate alternative etiologies such as calciphylaxis, pyoderma gangrenosum, or sickle cell disease. In addition to arterial and venous disease, the differential diagnosis also includes diabetic neuropathic ulcer, pressure ulcer, vasculitis, infection, malignancies, or trauma. Diagnosis frequently requires a comprehensive assessment of the medical history, physical exam, laboratory tests, imaging studies, and sometimes wound biopsy. With VLUs, a physical exam and venous reflux studies will most likely help confirm your diagnosis; however, additional contributing factors should also be ruled out.

Diagnostics

In our wound center, we utilize an algorithm for the workup and treatment of VLUs (Table 7.1). This includes ankle-brachial indices (ABIs) with toe pressure and pulse volume recordings (PVRs) to determine inflow and arterial status and to help guide the level of compression with concurrent mixed arterial and venous disease. Discordant ABIs or an index <9 in the affected limb warrants arterial duplex ultrasound.

Table 7.1 MGH lower extremity venous treatment algorithm

Full history and physical	
Photo of wound(s) with measurements	
Assess pulses, edema, skin color, temperature	
Signs and symptoms of infection:	NERDS (non-healing, exudate, red/friable, debris, smell) = *treat topically*
	STONES (size change, temperature, osteomyelitis, new skin breakdown, exudate/erythema/edema, smell) = *treat with systemic antibiotics*
Data: labs (including nutritional, inflammatory, Hemoglobin A1C), imaging	
Identify and address risk factors: immobility, history of trauma, DVT, congenital venous abnormality, CHF, age	
Characteristic presentation: hemosiderin staining, lipodermatosclerosis, varicosities, dermatitis, location.	

Toe blood pressure is beneficial when ABI is nondiagnostic, as commonly seen in the elderly and in patients with DM due to the hardening of the blood vessel walls. Toe blood pressure <30 mmHg has been associated with a non-healing relative risk of 3.25 (95% CI 1.96–5.41). Although this is true for arterial ulcers, it also stands true with mixed ulcers with a venous and arterial components of disease [1, 2]. Venous duplex and reflux studies are warranted, as well as a referral to vascular surgery for possible surgical intervention if deemed to be a good candidate.

Wound cultures, either swab or tissue, are not routinely performed on a chronic wound without signs of acute infection. Tissue biopsy is typically indicated for non-healing wounds greater than 6 months, particularly if they are in an atypical location.

Management

If the underlying etiology of the wound is surgically correctable or can be surgically improved, this should be performed in parallel with appropriate non-surgical treatments. In addition, it is essential to address and acknowledge the patient's risk factors for delayed healing, i.e., poor nutritional status, obesity, diabetes, comorbidities, immunosuppression, or smoking. As with all wounds, the principles of effective wound care include debridement of devitalized tissue, decreasing bioburden, optimizing perfusion, optimizing moisture balance, and prompt wound closure.

Debridement

Sharp debridement is one component used to optimize the wound environment. Sharp debridement of a chronic wound, particularly in the context of a VLU, offers several advantages: removal of nonviable tissue, decreased bioburden, disruption of biofilm, removal of slough and eschar, reduced infectious risk, improved efficacy of topical treatments, enhanced pain management, allows for accurate assessment of wound depth and extent, and ultimately promotes healing and reduces time to wound closure. Other forms of debridement include enzymatic, mechanical, autolytic, and chemical (absorbent sodium chloride-impregnated dressing).

Topical Wound Care

For those presenting with signs of local infection (non-healing, increased exudate, red/friable tissue, increased debris, malodor), it is appropriate to treat them with topical antiseptics.

Topical wound care is used to address bioburden, as well as for exudate management and patient comfort. For locally infected wounds or surrounding cellulitis, options include sodium hypochlorite solution (0.125% strength) or hypochlorous solution applied to gauze covered with an absorbent dressing. Antiseptic silver options are available in alginate, hydrofiber, and foam for absorbent products. Cadexomer iodine is also an effective broad-spectrum antiseptic. Note that we are very cautious in using antiseptics but not topical antibiotics, as the latter have not been shown to reduce the risk of wound infections and are associated with antibiotic resistance and, in some instances, impaired wound healing [3]. For wounds with overlying eschar in patients where sharp excision is not performed, sulfamylon cream, silver sulfadiazine cream, or wound gel can facilitate autolytic debridement. Large wounds with slough/devitalized tissue and high-volume exudate benefit from a hypertonic, impregnated, nonwoven-type dressing that will clean and absorb. Most venous ulcers have moderate to large amounts of exudate, so an absorbent product is typically utilized. Dressing products such as alginates, hydrofibers, cadexomer iodine, foams, and hydroconductive pads can also be used. If the patient experiences pain with dressing removal due to product adherence, a silicone open-weave contact layer can first be placed on the wound bed, followed by the secondary dressing.

The patient requires systemic antibiotics if there are signs of cellulitis or systemic infection (increased size, fever, new bone exposure, increased exudate, erythema/cellulitis, edema, or odor).

Peri-wound Skin Management

Peri-wound skin management is essential due to the risk of denudement and skin breakdown from a highly exudative ulcer. Skin protection can be achieved using acrylate or cyanoacrylate skin barrier films (wipes or spray) or barrier creams (dimethicone, zinc, petroleum, or similar). Occasionally, a short course of topical steroids can also be used to treat a surrounding dermatitis.

Compression

Compression is a critical element of venous ulcer care. At a tissue level, compression therapy increases interstitial pressure, reducing fluid filtration from the venous capillaries and improving venous pumping function. At a cellular level, it has been postulated to decrease inflammatory cytokines, immune complex adhesion, and extravasation.

Although most current guidelines recommend maximum compression, ABIs should first be used to evaluate for peripheral arterial disease and guide the compression strength (Tables 7.2 and 7.3). Compression therapy promotes arterial flow and microcircu-

Table 7.2 Lower extremity compression

High 30+ mmHg ABI ≥0.8	*Medium* 20–30 mmHg ABI 0.5–0.8	*Light* 15–20 mmHg ABI <0.5	*Little* <15 mmHg
Profore	Profore light	One layer tubigrip	ACE wrap
Coban 2 layer	Unna's boot	TED stockings	
Setopress or Surepress			

Table 7.3 Choice of compression

Elastic and gradient wraps	Profore Coban—2 Profore—light
Inelastic wrap	Unna's boot Short stretch wrap, as used in lymphedema management
Long-term therapy	Inelastic velcro wraps (circaids, FarrowWrap, etc.) Compressions stockings Intermittent pneumatic pumps

lation, provided that compression pressure remains lower than the intra-arterial pressure. While lighter compression therapies may be used on patients with ABIs of <0.5 and absolute systolic ankle pressure >60 mmHg, we prioritize arterial revascularization in such cases.

Long-term compression therapy is an essential component of the successful treatment of venous ulcerations and limits recurrence. However, compliance with compression therapy can be challenging. Its value should be carefully explained to patients so that they can embrace this treatment/prevention modality and commit to lifelong application. For the patients who have never used compression, we found a graduated approach to be more successful. Start with low pressure and advance until full compression is achieved. First-line compression options include elastic tubular bandaging or an open-weave design. This can be advanced to a graduated compression wrap or multilayer compression dressing (Fig. 7.2). The amount of exudate may also impact the selected type of compression. For example, a large and

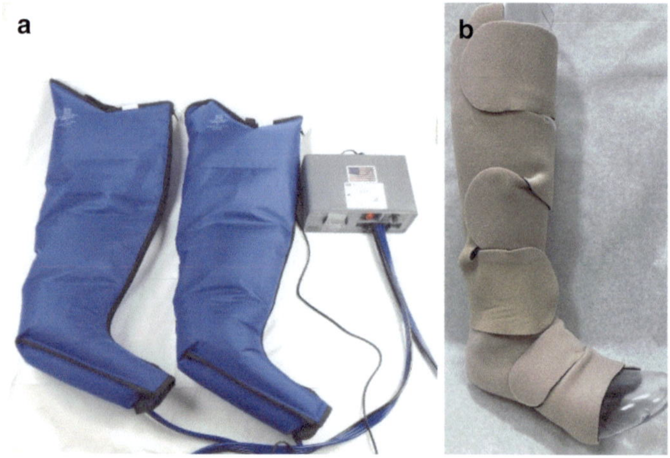

Fig. 7.2 (**a**) Pneumatic pump. (**b**) Velcro-style compression garment

highly exudative ulcer would be appropriate for an absorbent dressing product and a graduated compression wrap that is easily applied and amenable to more frequent dressing changes. A lower-exudative ulcer would be more amenable to a topical dressing with a multilayer compression wrap and less frequent changes. Long-term compression options include 30–40 mm Hg compression hose, Velcro-style wrap garments, and pneumatic compression pumps (Fig. 7.3).

Physical therapy is also critical to help increase ambulation and obtain a full range of motion at the knee and ankle in order to optimize the use of the calf muscle pump for venous return. Lastly, pain should be adequately treated so that the patient can fully participate in the plan of care, including compression and topical wound care (Figs. 7.4 and 7.5).

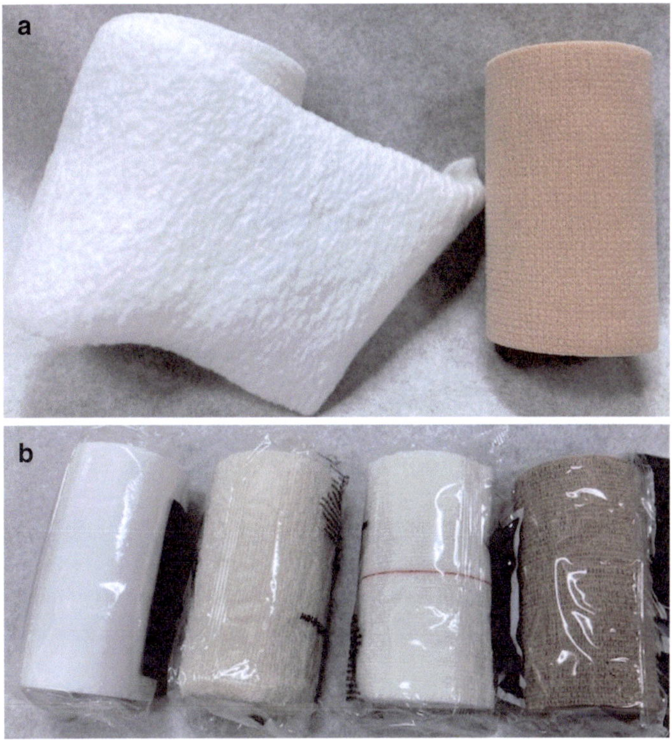

Fig. 7.3 (**a**) Two-layer wrap. (**b**) Four-layer wrap

Surgical Management

Negative Pressure Wound Therapy (NPWT)

Negative pressure wound therapy (NPWT) is an excellent option to treat VLUs as it manages exudate, promotes wound contraction, and stimulates granulation formation. We frequently use NPWT after sharp debridement to prepare the wound bed for split-thickness skin grafting (STSG). Depending on the patient and the wound size, STSGs can be performed in the OR or in the treatment room of our outpatient clinic.

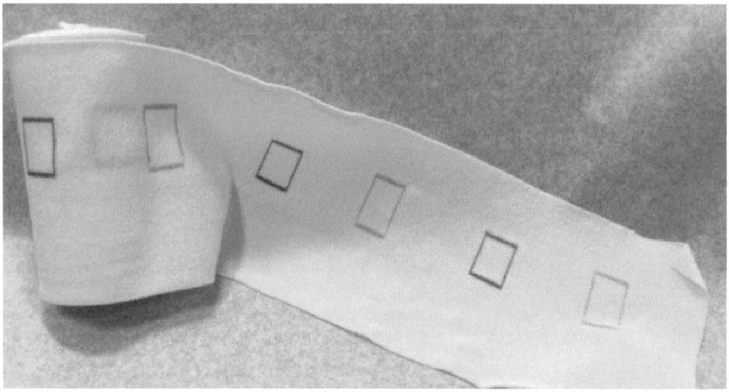

Fig. 7.4 Graduated compression

Placental-Based Allografts and Split-Thickness Skin Grafting (STSG)

Optimally, wound bed preparation includes surgical debridement in the clinic followed by at least 1 week of NPWT. The following is our note template detailing the procedure and post-op management:

Procedure Note for STSG Performed in the Clinic

Excisional debridement surgical prep of wound to Right Foot with Right thigh donor site.

Diagnosis: Chronic wound to Right foot.

Procedural/Surgical Consent obtained.

Time out: Immediately prior to the procedure, a time out was called. A time-out verifies the correct patient, procedure, equipment, support staff, and site/side marked as required.

30 cc of 1% lidocaine was used to anesthetize the area of the right thigh donor site and right foot. The right thigh and right lower leg were prepped and draped in a sterile fashion.

Excisional debridement/surgical prep to wound bed performed with pressure and gauze for hemostasis.

A 2-inch guard and a 12-inch/1000th-inch Zimmer are used to harvest donor skin.

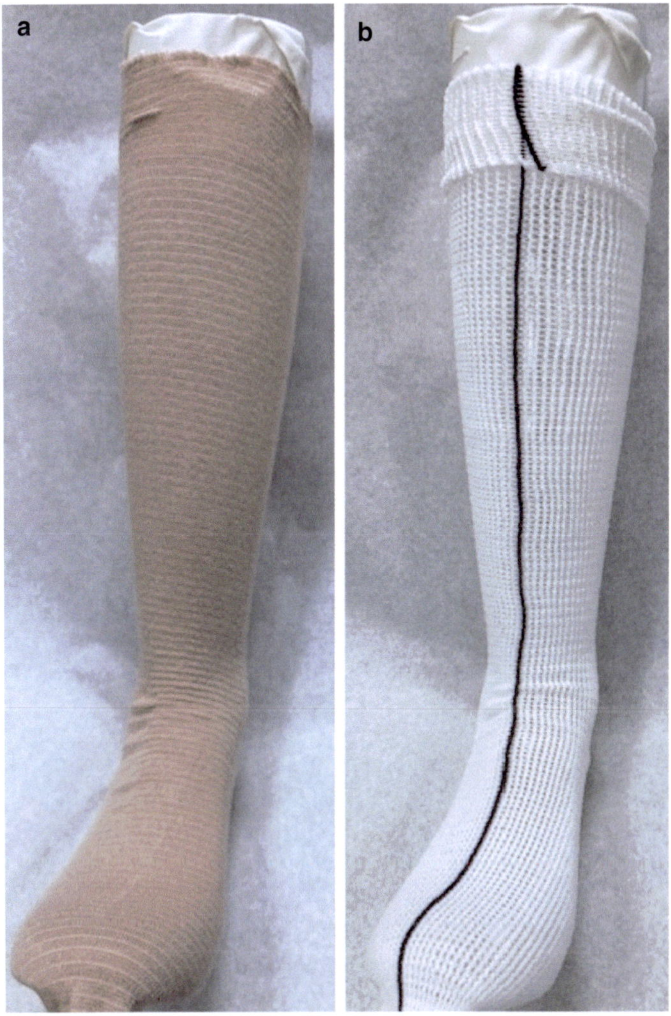

Fig. 7.5 (**a**) Elastic tubular stocking. (**b**) Open weave wale stocking

Meshed with 1:1 mesher.
Applied to wound bed with staples.
Mepilex AG stapled to donor and wrapped with Kerlix and Coban.
Bactroban, adaptic, kerlix, ACE wrap applied.
No acute complications were noted.
Follow-up in 5 days for removal of bolster in clinic.

Follow-Up for STSG of Wound Patients

No dressing changes until the first follow-up in 5 days.
Donor site Mepilex Ag removed and fresh Mepilex Ag applied for another 5–7 days.
Graft site typically treated with daily or QOD Bactroban or Bacitracin, Adaptic, and DSD.
The next follow-up is in 7 days, at which time the donor and graft sites receive Bactroban or Bacitracin, Adpatic, and DSD daily or QOD.
Typically healed by 2–3 weeks and then move to moisturizer only.
Occasionally, 3–5 days of topically high-potency steroid ointment is used to treat inflammation or hypergranulation at the graft or donor site.

Venous Interventions

- ESCHAR Study (2004): Effect of surgery and compression on ulcer healing and recurrence
- EVRA Study (2018): Early Venous Reflux Ablation in venous ulceration

In 2004, the Effect of Surgery and Compression on Healing and Recurrence (ESCHAR) study randomized 500 subjects with venous insufficiency and venous ulcers to compression with and without surgery. Overall, ulcer healing rates did not reach a statistically significant difference at 3 years. However, upon healing, ulcer recurrence rates were significantly lower in the compression plus surgery group compared with the compression group (31% vs. 56%; $P < 0.001$).

With the advent of new venous intervention techniques and anecdotic experience showing improved ulcer healing rates, the Early Venous Reflux Ablation in venous ulceration (EVRA) study attempted to challenge the ESCHAR results by stratifying patients to early intervention (ulcers <6 months) versus deferred intervention. The results of this study sedimented the importance of early treatment of venous disease in these patients. The median time to ulcer healing was 56 days (95% CI 49–66) in the early intervention group and 82 days (95% CI 69–92) in the deferred intervention group.

How Do We Define a Healing Wound?

A healing wound is defined by a decrease in objective measurements of size, with a goal of at least a 20% reduction after 2 weeks of treatment. In addition to size, healing is also noted by the presence of healthy, beefy-red, granulating tissue, clean serous or serosanguinous exudate, decreasing exudate, lack of odor, and epithelialization from the wound edges. Our wound center regularly uses split-thickness skin grafting to facilitate and expedite wound closure. Factors to consider concerning surgical wound closure (i.e., STSG) include large surface area (>100 cm^2), pain with dressings, or the need for expedited healing in order to address other issues (e.g., immunosuppression or a patient requiring wound closure in order to have surgery for another condition).

Complications and Management

The most common complications we see in treating venous ulcers include wound infection, cellulitis, and failure to achieve wound closure. Wound infection is typically treated with surgical excision under local anesthesia or in the operating room. The goal is to achieve source control by removing all devitalized tissue. Cellulitis is treated with oral or IV antibiotics. The reason is often multifactorial when a wound fails to heal with appropriate treatment, as outlined above. It is often reasonable to re-establish the diagnosis and obtain a punch biopsy to ensure no other factors are involved in the etiology of the wound. A short trial (3–5 days) of a high-potency topical steroid may also be appropriate.

If a STSG fails to close a wound in ~4–6 weeks, we consider this a skin graft failure and try something else. A different topical, a more aggressive debridement, or NPWT with or without a dermal matrix (Integra or BTM) followed by another attempt at STSG. Local flaps or even free tissue transfer are additional options.

Key Point Synopsis

Establishing the diagnosis with an appropriate workup.

Fix the underlying problems if possible.

Healing venous ulceration requires not only treatment of the wound but also the treatment of the patient attached to the wound. Patient treatment frequently entails lifestyle modification and compliance; therefore, patient education is critical.

Plan per Primary Team

- Antibiotics
- Management of comorbid conditions (DM, renal, resp, CHF, etc.)
- Pain management

Orders

- X-ray, CT, or MRI to r/o osteomyelitis
- Inflammatory markers
- Nutrition labs (albumin, prealbumin, transferrin, H/H, and other labs as deemed pertinent)
- Arterial lower extremity non-invasive tests
- Venous duplex and reflux studies
- Vascular surgery consult, as indicated

Wound Service Plan

- OR vs. bedside debridement: Urgent OR in case of extensive wounds, immunocompromised, or systemic symptoms (fever, leukocytosis, altered mental status, hypotension, tachycardia)
- IV antibiotics for associated cellulitis
- Topical wound care and treat dermatitis, if present
- If large or long-term, consider wound bed prep with NPWT followed by STSG
- Debride chronic wounds to reduce biofilm (chronic, no progress 2 weeks, signs and symptoms of inflammation)
- Initiate compression and titrate up; use bedside pneumatic pumps
- Cultures, Wound biopsy as needed
- Identify and control causative/contributing factors: DVT, tobacco use, obesity, sedentary.
- Patient evaluation and treatment to improve mobility and increase ambulation
- Vascular surgery outpatient referral, venous duplex studies

DVT: deep venous thrombosis; CHF: congestive heart failure; H/H: hemoglobin/hematocrit; OR: operating room; NPWT: negative pressure wound therapy; STSG: split thickness skin graft

Summary

Venous leg ulcers are open wounds that typically develop on the lower legs, often near the ankles (gaiter areas), due to poor circulation and vein dysfunction. They are commonly associated with chronic venous insufficiency (CVI), a condition in which the veins in the legs are unable to effectively return blood to the heart. As blood pools in the veins, increased pressure and local chronic hypoxia can damage the skin and tissues, leading to the formation of ulcers. The primary risk factors for venous leg ulcers include age, obesity, prolonged standing, a history of deep vein thrombosis (DVT), and a family history of venous disease. Symptoms include pain, swelling, and redness around the ulcer, and the wound often has a wet or weeping appearance due to fluid buildup. The ulcers are usually slow to heal and may be recurrent. Management focuses on improving circulation, controlling symptoms, and promoting healing. This typically involves compression therapy (to reduce swelling and improve blood flow), wound care, and sometimes medications to manage infection or inflammation. In the setting of superficial venous insufficiency, minimally invasive surgical intervention may be needed to accelerate the healing process and prevent recurrence.

References

1. Sonter JA, Ho A, Chuter VH. The predictive capacity of toe blood pressure and the toe brachial index for foot wound healing and amputation: a systematic review and meta-analysis. Wound Pract Res. 2014;22(4):208.
2. Mosti G, Iabichella ML, Partsch H. Compression therapy in mixed ulcers increases venous output and arterial perfusion. J Vasc Surg. 2012;55(1):122–8. https://doi.org/10.1016/j.jvs.2011.07.071. ISSN 0741-5214.
3. Fathy R, Chu B, Singh P, James WD, Barbieri JS. Variation in topical antibiotics recommendations in wound care instructions by non-dermatologists. J Gen Intern Med. 2020;36(1):238–9. https://doi.org/10.1007/s11606-020-05689-2.

Suggested Reading

Hess CT. Venous ulcer assessment and management: using the updated CEAP classification system. Adv Skin Wound Care. 2020;33(11):614–5. https://doi.org/10.1097/01.ASW.0000719052.33284.73.

Kelechi TJ, Brunette G, Bonham PA, Crestodina L, Droste LR, Ratliff CR, Varnado MF. 2019 Guideline for management of wounds in patients with lower-extremity venous disease (LEVD). An executive summary. J Wound Ostomy Continence Nurs. 2020;47(2):97–110. https://doi.org/10.1097/WON.0000000000000622.

Millan SB, Gan R, Townsend PE. Venous ulcers: diagnosis and treatment. Am Fam Physician. 2019;100(5):298–305. Accessed 7 Aug 2023. https://search-ebscohost-com.treadwell.idm.oclc.org/login.aspx?direct=true&db=mdc&AN=EPTOC138405097&site=ehost-live&scope=site.

Snyder RJ, Jensen J, Applewhite AJ, Couch K, Joseph WS, Lantis Ii JC, Serena TE. A standardized approach to evaluating lower extremity chronic wounds using a checklist. Wounds Compend Clin Res Pract. 2019;31(5 Suppl):S29–44. Retrieved from https://phstwlp2.partners.org:3700/login.aspx?direct=true&db=mdc&AN=31033453&site=eds-live&scope=site.

O'Donnell TF, Passman MA, Marston WA, Ennis WJ, Dalsing M, Kistner RL, Lurie F, Henke PK, Gloviczki ML, Eklöf BG, Stoughton J, Raju S, Shortell CK, Raffetto JD, Partsch H, Pounds LC, Cummings ME, Gillespie DL, McLafferty RB, Murad MH, Wakefield TW, Gloviczki P. Management of venous leg ulcers: clinical practice guidelines of the Society for Vascular Surgery® and the American Venous Forum. J Vasc Surg. 2014;60(2 Suppl):3S–59S. https://doi.org/10.1016/j.jvs.2014.04.049. ISSN 0741-5214. https://www.sciencedirect.com/science/article/pii/S0741521414008519.

Neurological Considerations for the Vein Specialist

8

Carlos Echevarria and Reza Seyedsadjadi

Case/Teaser

A 57-year-old female was referred to neurology for evaluation of significant pain, numbness, and tingling in the dorsum and bottom of her left foot, alongside weakness in ankle plantar flexion. She had a past medical history of superficial venous insufficiency and underwent radiofrequency ablation of her left great saphenous vein right before the onset of symptoms. Imaging revealed deep vein thrombosis in the popliteal vein, extending to complete occlusion of the femoral vein, for which she is currently on apixaban.

A detailed motor exam revealed weakness primarily in plantar flexion, toe flexion, and foot inversion. Deep tendon

C. Echevarria (✉)
Division of Vascular and Endovascular Surgery, Department of Surgery, Massachusetts General Hospital/Harvard Venous & Lymphatic Medicine Alumni, Boston, MA, USA

Division of Vascular Medicine and Endovenous Interventions, Veins & Vascular Centers of Excellence, Phoenix, AZ, USA
e-mail: carlos.echevarria@vascular.md

R. Seyedsadjadi
Department of Neurology – Neuromuscular Medicine, Massachusetts General Hospital/Harvard Medical School, Boston, MA, USA
e-mail: rseyedsadjadi@mgh.harvard.edu

C. Echevarria et al. (eds.), *The Massachusetts General Hospital Protocols and Procedures for Venous Disease*,
https://doi.org/10.1007/978-3-032-05708-2_8

reflexes were diminished at the left ankle. The sensory exam was notable for reduced sensation to pinprick stimuli in the bottom of the left foot.

Anatomy of the Disease

When it comes to neurological pathology associated with venous disease, it is essential first to characterize chronicity and locate the underlying process. Recognizing major neuroanatomical associations in the lower extremities is important to avoid complications associated with venous insufficiency procedures. In brief, the lumbosacral nerve roots (L2–S2) give branches to two major plexi (Fig. 8.1):

1. Lumbar plexus (L2–L4) branching to femoral (hip flexion and knee extension) and obturator nerves (hip adduction).
2. Lumbosacral plexus (L5–S2) branching to gluteal (gluteus maximus and medius) and sciatic nerves. Sciatic nerve branches to peroneal and tibial divisions.

Femoral Nerve

The femoral nerve runs behind the inguinal ligament, entering the femoral triangle and traveling through the adductor canal. It provides motor function to the front thigh muscles, controlling hip flexion and knee extension. In terms of sensory function, it branches into anterior cutaneous branches, which supply sensory function to the anterior and medial surface of the thigh.

The saphenous nerve, an extension of the posterior division of the femoral nerve, is responsible for sensory supply to the skin of the medial leg and foot. The saphenous nerve runs along the femoral artery and vein within the adductor canal, later traveling more medial and superficial along the great saphenous vein right below the knee. Although difficult to visualize with ultrasound, local anesthetic along a transverse line between the medial femoral epicondyles is the preferred method utilized for

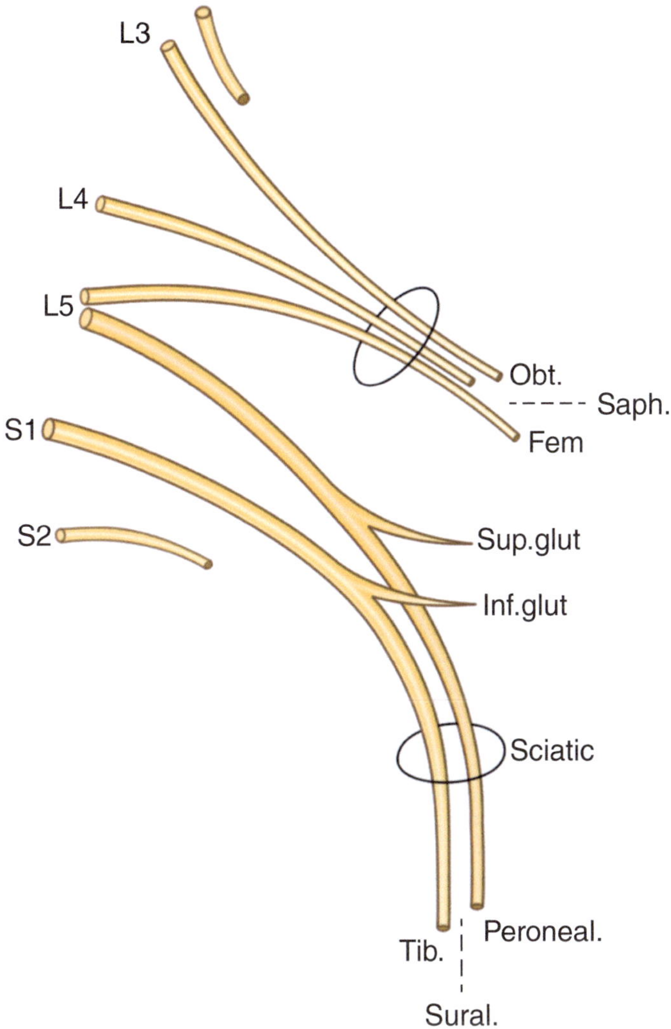

Fig. 8.1 The lumbosacral nerve roots (L2–S2). Obt: Obturator nerve (hip adduction); fem: femoral nerve (hip flexion and knee extension); Saph: saphenous nerve (sensory); tib: tibial nerve (plantar flexion and foot inversion and sensory branches); sural nerve (sensory); Peroneal (sensory)

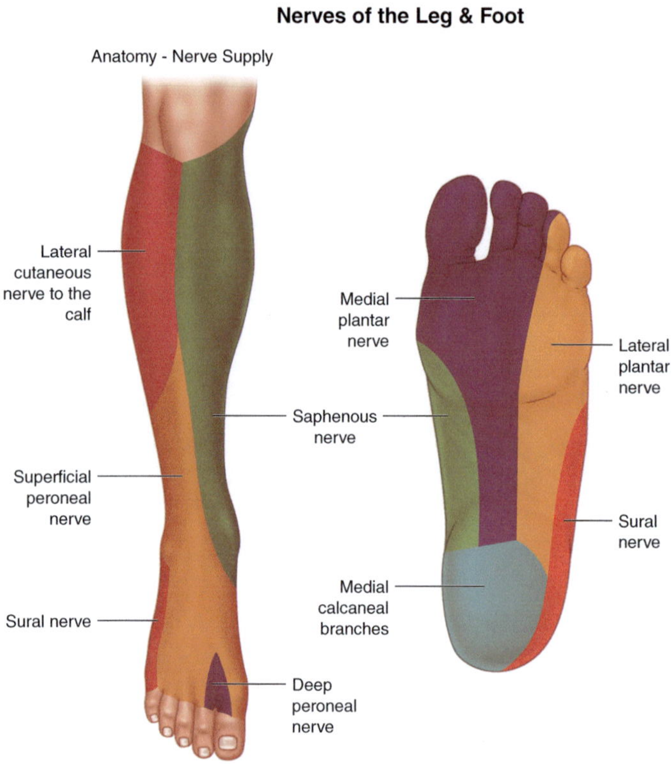

Fig. 8.2 Sensory nerve distribution below the knee. GSV thermal ablation may affect the saphenous nerve (green) due to its proximity to the vein when running below the knee. Similarly, the SSV runs along the sural nerve (red). A precise tumescent technique can separate these elements to avoid complications

a saphenous nerve block in this region [1]. This effect may also be unintendedly achieved with local anesthetic for the treatment of a distal calf pathological perforator (Cocket I), when tumescent anesthesia extends 1–2 cm superior and anterior to the medial malleolus [2, 3] (Fig. 8.2).

Sciatic Nerve

After its formation from the pelvic region, the sciatic nerve gains access to the gluteal area by passing through the greater sciatic foramen. The sciatic nerve directly controls the muscles situated in the posterior thigh compartment. An ultrasound probe placed in the transverse position over the apex of the popliteal fossa will show the sciatic nerve division into the tibial and common peroneal trunks.

The tibial nerve governs the calf muscles (plantar flexion and foot inversion) and controls specific intrinsic foot muscles. The tibial nerve supplies the posterolateral leg's sensory function, the foot's lateral aspect via its sural nerve branches, and the sole via terminal branches. When fanning the ultrasound probe over the popliteal fossa, the tibial nerve can be seen as a round echogenic structure between the popliteal and small saphenous vein. In a longitudinal view, the tibial nerve runs along and superficial to the popliteal vein [4].

The sural nerve, responsible for sensory functions in the lower leg, is formed by branches originating mainly from the tibial and peroneal nerves. It runs parallel and near the small saphenous vein. The sural nerve provides sensory innervation to the lower half posterolateral aspect of the calf and the lateral section of the dorsum of the foot and 5th toe.

The common peroneal nerve (common fibular) governs the anterior and lateral leg muscles and the remaining intrinsic foot muscles. The common peroneal nerve handles sensory innervation for the skin of the lateral leg and the dorsum of the foot. This nerve becomes more superficial when running to the lateral aspect of the fibular head. This predisposes the peroneal nerve to trauma.

Mononeuropathies are unilateral and follow individual nerve patterns. In contrast, more than a third of patients with venous insufficiency may present with paresthesias, often bilateral [5]. There is an association between the degree of peripheral neuropathy and venous disease burden [6]. It has been hypothesized that chronic venous insufficiency may trigger microangiopathic changes leading to skin changes and paresthesias. Neuropathic symptom distribution correlates with skin trophic changes. Similarly, lower extremity edema and venous stasis may lead to diminished sensation in the lower extremities and may not necessarily follow a specific nerve pathway [7].

Differential Diagnosis

The most common differential for the vascular specialist is arterial and venous disease. Assessment of risk factors such as tobacco and diabetes, along with symptoms associated with claudication, should precede any further tests. A 2-point ankle-brachial index may aid in the detection of peripheral arterial disease. Venous symptomatology, such as heaviness, aching, and throbbing pain, may be interpreted as neurological symptoms. Venous insufficiency, venous compression syndromes, and superficial thrombophlebitis should be considered in the differential diagnosis of peripheral neuropathy.

Although uncommon, sciatic pain may be triggered by superficial varicosities along the sciatic and tibial nerves. Unlike lumbosacral radiculopathy, leg elevation tends to improve venous symptoms. Recommendations for sciatic nerve pain may sometimes overlap with those offered for venous disease, such as avoiding the sitting position for prolonged periods and ambulation [8].

Restless leg syndrome may mimic or even exacerbate vascular or neurological symptoms. It is, however, a different entity and will require a diagnostic journey to rule out other etiologies. As a stand-alone condition, restless leg symptoms are typically worse at rest with at least temporary relief with activity, similar to venous pathology, so vascular studies are warranted. Studies have shown improvement in restless leg symptoms with venous interventions [9]. Positive (burning, tingling) or negative (numbness) sensory symptoms are not typical but may concur.

Baker's cysts are a common non-vascular finding during venous duplex examination. Due to the absence of structural support from the synovial capsule, they predominantly develop in the posteromedial region of the popliteal fossa. However, when growing larger, Baker's cysts may expand toward the posterolateral side, leading to the compression of the tibial nerve. This could potentially result in tibial neuropathy as a possible manifestation [10].

There is a broad differential diagnosis for polyneuropathy. In general, neuropathies can be grouped into three categories: (1) acquired; associated with systemic diseases, diabetes mellitus, proteinopathies, toxic (e.g., ethanol), inflammatory, infectious, nutritional, and vasculitic processes; (2) hereditary; Charcot-Marie-Tooth disease, Fabry disease, etc.; and (3) idiopathic, when there is no clear explanation for neuropathy. The latter is commonly present in adults >50 years of age and has an insidious progression of typically sensory symptoms [11, 12].

Diagnostics/Auxilliary Testing/Imaging Studies

A comprehensive clinical history and neurological examination usually deliver an accurate diagnosis. Any history of trauma or prior interventions should be thoroughly assessed. Ankle reflex is a sensitive diagnostic tool, easily performed in the outpatient setting. The exam can be further improved when combined with pinprick or vibratory stimuli [13] (Tables 8.1 and 8.2).

Table 8.1 Mononeuropathies

Roots	Nerve	Motor	Sensory
L2–L4	Femoral	Hip flexion Knee extension	Anterior thigh Medial calf
L2–L4	Obturator	Hip adduction	Medial thigh
L2–L4	Saphenous	–	Medial calf
L4–S3	Sciatic	Knee flexion Ankle dorsiflexion Plantar flexion Foot eversion and inversion	Lateral calf foot
L4–S1	Peroneal	Ankle dorsiflexion Foot eversion	Dorsum of the foot
L5–S3	Tibial	Plantar flexion Foot inversion	Bottom of the foot
L4–S3	Sural	–	Posterior/lateral calf and foot

Table 8.2 Nerve roots

Roots	Nerve	Motor	Sensory
L3/S4		Hip flexion Hip adduction Knee extension	Thigh Medial calf
L5	Obturator	Hip abduction Ankle dorsiflexion Foot inversion	Lateral calf
S1	Saphenous	Hip extension Knee flexion Plantar flexion Foot inversion	Bottom of the foot

Auxilliary Testing/Imaging Studies

Chronic venous insufficiency may present concurrently with many of the conditions described above, making the diagnosis uncertain and the treatment outcome difficult to predict. Although it is essential to partner with a neurologist, the venous specialist should know what to expect from a neurology evaluation. Patients should be evaluated initially for common etiologies associated with acquired neuropathies, i.e., diabetes and proteinopathies. Initial laboratory testing with the highest detection yield are HemoglobinA1c, folic acid, vitamin B12, methylmalonic acid, and serum/urine protein immunofixation electrophoresis (SPEP/UPEP) studies [14].

Duplex and soft tissue ultrasound is a fast and inexpensive image modality that can rule out other pathologies, including Baker's cyst. Varicosities along the sciatic and tibial nerves are not necessarily associated with saphenous or deep vein reflux [15]; therefore, placing the ultrasound probe on the back of the leg may render an immediate diagnosis.

Focused neuromuscular examination and neurophysiology (electromyography and nerve conduction studies) are typically employed when the cause is uncertain and can help localize and characterize the neurogenic process. Electromyography (EMG) studies are warranted to evaluate axonal continuity in more severe pathologies. We often rely on functional neurophysiology to differentiate between preganglionic (radiculopathy or segmental myelopathy) and postganglionic (plexus or peripheral nerve) processes. A multifocal process raises clinician suspicion for a more generalized condition such as mononeuritis multiplex (affects two or more non-continuous nerves) or acquired demyelinating neuropathies.

Skin biopsy may, at times, be helpful in the diagnosis of small fiber neuropathy. Nerve biopsy is seldom used to identify the root cause of polyneuropathy unless vasculitis is suspected.

Management

Medical Management

For patients with polyneuropathy, any minor unattended trauma may become an ulcer, as patients have lost their primary signal of pain. With it, they have also lost the motivation to take care of it.

Up to 20–25% of patients with diabetes will develop a foot ulcer due to peripheral neuropathy, and this risk significantly increases to over 50% in those with a prior history of wounds [16]. Compression is one of the pillars of conservative management for chronic wounds and chronic venous insufficiency. Patients with polyneuropathy, however, may feel an exacerbation of their symptoms. I have found aquatherapy to be a beneficial alternative, as water pressure may replicate the effect of compression stockings (water pressure is equivalent to 76 mmHg every 3 feet underwater).

Addressing the underlying etiology is the mainstay of treatment. Gabapentinoids and antidepressants, including duloxetine and tricyclic antidepressants, are often prescribed to alleviate polyneuropathy-related symptoms and are typically well tolerated. Physicians should refrain from employing opioids in the treatment of painful diabetic neuropathy [17]. A short course of steroids may help with short-term inflammatory processes.

Endovascular/Surgical Interventions

The etiology of the condition will guide therapy. Regardless, patients often describe improvement in their polyneuropathy symptoms after superficial venous ablation interventions.

Regarding venous-associated neuropathies, direct intervention to refluxing veins and venous varicosities along the sciatic and tibial nerves have shown significant improvement and even complete resolution of signs and symptoms [15]. Caution must be taken with ablation method selection to avoid further nerve damage.

Surveillance

The venous specialist must consider the new patient's baseline for further interventions.

In addition to specific treatments for the common processes associated with acquired neuropathies, we often refer patients to physical therapy for core strength and balance.

Complications and Management

Complications of Thermal Ablation

The saphenous nerve is predominantly sensory. It runs parallel along the distal portion of the great saphenous vein (GSV) below the knee. Caution must be taken when performing thermal ablation near or below the knee, as damage to the saphenous nerve may result in sensory loss to the medial aspect of the calf. Due to this common complication, it is now the standard of care to avoid thermal ablation of the GSV at or below the knee level. Despite caution, up to 15% of patients may report some degree of post-op neuropathy, with most cases resolving over 2 years [18].

The tibial nerve's deeper positioning makes it less susceptible to injury during phlebectomy. However, when passing through the popliteal fossa, it is close to the sapheno-popliteal Junction (SPJ), facing potential risk during endovenous thermal ablation procedures [19]. In the event of injury, manifestations often include an inability to perform plantar flexion and sensory deficits affecting the sole of the foot.

The sural nerve runs along the Small Saphenous Vein (SSV), and although its course is highly variable, they remain within 5 mm from each other. To minimize the risk of nerve damage, the ideal location for endovenous ablation of the SSV is in the upper one-third of the leg, where a natural fascial barrier exists between the SSV and the sural nerve. The risk is heightened when tumescent anesthesia is insufficient in the lower two-thirds of the leg due to their proximity and the absence of deep fascia between these structures [19].

Neurological Complications of Phlebectomy

The common peroneal nerve is one of two terminal branches of the sciatic nerve. It courses along the medial head of the biceps femoris tendon and traverses the lateral aspect of the fibular head, where it can be injured during phlebectomy. Injury to the nerve typically results in foot drop and sensory loss to the dorsal surface of the foot and portions of the anterolateral aspect of the lower leg.

Sural nerve lesion has also been reported as a complication of phlebectomy. This is due to its superficial anatomy in the posterior calf [20]. To avoid neurological complications, the physician must reconsider their approach at any sign of pain.

It is commonly observed in clinical practice that paresthesias tend to get better over time for most patients. Nonetheless, it is undeniable that a minority of patients may progress to experience a highly distressing dysesthetic pain syndrome.

The true incidence of neurological complications is unknown, as most physicians are reluctant to publish negative outcome data. Therefore, it is unclear if neurological complications are just collateral damage or constitute an actual breach of duty. As a result, it is essential to discuss these risks in detail with patients.

Forensic Analysis: Dissecting the Case

The case described at the beginning of this chapter presented for treatment of superficial venous insufficiency of the GSV. Instead, the interventionalist probably accessed the popliteal vein and ablated the femoral vein distal to the profunda femoris, possibly confounding it with the saphenofemoral junction. For this to happen, I suspect the interventionalist inadvertently collapsed the GSV when placing the ultrasound probe over the leg, exposing the femoral vein as the largest vessel that runs along the medial thigh. This is particularly common in patients with low BMI, such as this case. Unable to distinguish it from any other more superficial vein, he proceeded with access and tumescent anesthesia, further clouding the picture. The GSV will usually be within the fascia, on what is described as the “Egyptian eye” for its resemblance to the Eye of Horus. The femoral vein runs along the femoral artery and nerve within the adductor canal. This case highlights the importance of acquiring the technical expertise and proper anatomical identification of all structures via ultrasound.

MRI showed thickening of the tibial nerve at the intercondylar notch with adjacent edema, which explains her inability to flex her foot and all the other neurological findings compatible with this type of injury. As the tibial nerve runs in close proximity to the popliteal vein, the unintended thermal ablation of this vein may have caused nerve injury and consequential complications.

Summary

Recognizing major neuroanatomical associations in the lower extremities is extremely important to avoid complications associated with venous insufficiency procedures. The saphenous nerve could be inadvertently blocked with the tumescent anesthesia of a Cockett's I perforator. Most concerning, it could also be affected by thermal injury when ablating the GSV below the knee. The tibial and sural nerves are also exposed to thermal injury if anatomical landmarks are not considered when performing superficial venous thermal ablation procedures. The common peroneal nerve could potentially be at risk of trauma during microphlebectomy when running superficial to the lateral aspect of the fibular head. Conversely, direct intervention to refluxing veins and venous varicosities along the sciatic and tibial nerves has shown significant improvement in polyneuropathy symptoms.

References

1. Krombach J, Gray AT. Sonography for saphenous nerve block near the adductor canal. Reg Anesth Pain Med. 2007;32(4):369–70.
2. Marian AA, Ranganath Y, Bayman EO, Senasu J, Brennan TJ. A comparison of 2 ultrasound-guided approaches to the saphenous nerve block: adductor canal versus distal transsartorial: a prospective, randomized, blinded, noninferiority trial. Reg Anesth Pain Med. 2015;40(5):623–30. https://doi.org/10.1097/AAP.0000000000000277. PMID: 26110441.

3. Delbos A, Philippe M, Clément C, Olivier R, Coppens S. Ultrasound-guided ankle block. History revisited. Best Pract Res Clin Anaesthesiol. 2019;33(1):79–93.
4. Labropoulos N, Tassiopoulos AK, Gasparis AP, Phillips B, Pappas PJ. Veins along the course of the sciatic nerve. J Vasc Surg. 2009;49(3):690–6. https://doi.org/10.1016/j.jvs.2008.09.061.
5. Ba ̈thge A. Zur Korrelation phlebologischer Symptome mit neurophysiologischen Befunden bei Patienten mit chronischer veno ̈ser Insuffizienz. Thesis, Medizinische Akademie. Magdeburg, 1984.
6. Padberg FT, Maniker AH, Carmel G, Pappas PJ, Silva M, Hobson RW. Sensory impairment: a feature of chronic venous insufficiency. J Vasc Surg. 1999;30(5):836–43. https://doi.org/10.1016/s0741-5214(99)70008-x.
7. Yim E, Vivas A, Maderal A, Kirsner RS. Neuropathy and ankle mobility abnormalities in patients with chronic venous disease. JAMA Dermatol. 2014;150(4):385. https://doi.org/10.1001/jamadermatol.2013.6723.
8. Thiery L. La veine du nerf sciatique impact clinique et the'rapeutique. Phlebologie. 1988;41:687–9.
9. Hayes CA, Kingsley JR, Hamby KR, Carlow J. The effect of endovenous laser ablation on restless legs syndrome. Phlebology. 2008;23(3):112–7. https://doi.org/10.1258/phleb.2007.007051. PMID: 18467618.
10. Sanchez JE, Conkling N, Labropoulos N. Compression syndromes of the popliteal neurovascular bundle due to Baker cyst. J Vasc Surg. 2011;54(6):1821–9. https://doi.org/10.1016/j.jvs.2011.07.079. Epub 2011 Sep 29. PMID: 21958564.
11. Pasnoor M, Nascimento OJ, Trivedi J, Wolfe GI, Nations S, Herbelin L, de Freitas MG, Quintanilha G, Khan S, Dimachkie M, Barohn R. North America and South America (NA-SA) neuropathy project. Int J Neurosci. 2013;123(8):563–7. https://doi.org/10.3109/00207454.2013.782026. Epub 2013 Apr 17. PMID: 23461611.
12. Hanewinckel R, Drenthen J, van Oijen M, Hofman A, van Doorn PA, Ikram MA. Prevalence of polyneuropathy in the general middle-aged and elderly population. Neurology. 2016;87(18):1892–8. https://doi.org/10.1212/WNL.0000000000003293. Epub 2016 Sep 28. PMID: 27683845.
13. Abraham A, Alabdali M, Alsulaiman A, Albulaihe H, Breiner A, Katzberg HD, Aljaafari D, Lovblom LE, Bril V. The sensitivity and specificity of the neurological examination in polyneuropathy patients with clinical and electrophysiological correlations. PLoS One. 2017;12(3):e0171597. https://doi.org/10.1371/journal.pone.0171597. PMID: 28249029; PMCID: PMC5332032.
14. England JD, Gronseth GS, Franklin G, Carter GT, Kinsella LJ, Cohen JA, Asbury AK, Szigeti K, Lupski JR, Latov N, Lewis RA, Low PA, Fisher MA, Herrmann DN, Howard JF Jr, Lauria G, Miller RG, Polydefkis M,

Sumner AJ, American Academy of Neurology. Practice Parameter: evaluation of distal symmetric polyneuropathy: role of laboratory and genetic testing (an evidence-based review). Report of the American Academy of Neurology, American Association of Neuromuscular and Electrodiagnostic Medicine, and American Academy of Physical Medicine and Rehabilitation. Neurology. 2009;72(2):185–92. https://doi.org/10.1212/01.wnl.0000336370.51010.a1. Epub 2008 Dec 3. PMID: 19056666.

15. Thiery L. La veine du nerf sciatique impact clinique et thérapeutique. Phlebologie. 1988;41:687–9.
16. Lavery LA, Peters EJ, Williams JR, Murdoch DP, Hudson A, Lavery DC, International Working Group on the Diabetic Foot. Reevaluating the way we classify the diabetic foot: restructuring the diabetic foot risk classification system of the International Working Group on the Diabetic Foot. Diabetes Care. 2008;31(1):154–6. https://doi.org/10.2337/dc07-1302. Epub 2007 Oct 12. PMID: 17934155.
17. Price R, Smith D, Franklin G, et al. Oral and topical treatment of painful diabetic polyneuropathy: practice guideline update summary. Neurology. 2021;98(1):31–43. https://doi.org/10.1212/wnl.0000000000013038.
18. Weiß R, Weiss MA. Controlled radiofrequency endovenous occlusion using a unique radiofrequency catheter under duplex guidance to eliminate saphenous varicose vein reflux: a 2-year follow-up. Dermatologic Surg. 2002;28(1):38–42. https://doi.org/10.1046/j.1524-4725.2002.01188.x.
19. Kerver A, Arie, Theeuwes HP, et al. The surgical anatomy of the small saphenous vein and adjacent nerves in relation to endovenous thermal ablation. J Vasc Surg. 2012;56(1):181–8. https://doi.org/10.1016/j.jvs.2011.11.127.
20. Seror P. Atteinte du nerf sural (saphène externe) liée à une pathologie de la veine petite saphène. A propos de 5 cas [Sural nerve neuropathy (external saphenous) linked to a disease of the small saphenous vein. Apropos of 5 cases]. J Mal Vasc. 2000;25(2):128–31. French. PMID: 10804394.

Podiatric Considerations for the Vein Specialist

9

Sara Rose-Sauld and Carlos Echevarria

Case/Teaser

A 60-year-old female with a medical history of obesity and hypertension, employed as a cashier in a grocery store, has been experiencing a worsening of lower extremity pain and heaviness with known venous insufficiency. Including a comprehensive examination of her foot morphology in the physical assessment is crucial. A growing body of evidence demonstrates a correlation between venous disease, pes cavus foot types, and hypermobility. In such cases, conservative management should include not only compression therapy but also address the biomechanics of the foot and lower leg through orthotics and specific exercises.

S. Rose-Sauld (✉)
Department of Foot and Ankle Orthopedics, Massachusetts General Hospital/Harvard Medical School, Boston, MA, USA
e-mail: Srose-sauld@mgh.harvard.edu

C. Echevarria
Division of Vascular and Endovascular Surgery, Department of Surgery, Massachusetts General Hospital/Harvard Venous & Lymphatic Medicine Alumni, Boston, MA, USA

Division of Vascular Medicine and Endovenous Interventions, Veins & Vascular Centers of Excellence, Phoenix, AZ, USA
e-mail: carlos.echevarria@vascular.md

C. Echevarria et al. (eds.), *The Massachusetts General Hospital Protocols and Procedures for Venous Disease*,
https://doi.org/10.1007/978-3-032-05708-2_9

The Clinical Picture

Anatomy of Disease: Arch Type, Hypermobility, and the Correlation to Venous Disease

There is a growing body of evidence supporting the role of the "foot pump" in venous return, in addition to the well-established muscle pump activity of the calf. This chapter will delve into the influence of intrinsic foot muscles, deep fascia, and their likely correlation with foot types and venous diseases.

The Calf Pump

The foot houses 29 muscles, categorized into intrinsic and extrinsic muscles. Extrinsic muscles of the foot originate in the calf and insert into the foot. Examples include the posterior tibialis, peroneus longus, gastrocnemius, and soleus. They have larger muscle bellies in the lower leg and contribute to power for more significant foot movements at the ankle. Most importantly, for the purpose of this chapter, they serve as the main muscular pump for venous return. The veins of the leg traverse through the powerful musculature of the extrinsic muscles, with the calf being particularly strong. Here, pressures can reach as high as 200 mmHg, contributing to increased pressure throughout the lower extremity venous system [1].

The Foot Pump

Both types of muscles, intrinsic and extrinsic, are vital for normal gait and overall foot function. The deep plantar arch and the perforating veins course between and within the intrinsic musculature and their connecting fascia. Intrinsic muscles originating and inserting within the foot include the dorsal and plantar interosseus, lumbricals, and quadratus plantae. Their primary function is to stabilize the arch and facilitate toe movements.

Recent insights indicate that the foot operates somewhat differently from the lower leg. Unique regions, such as the heel, play a role in shunting blood proximally, medially, and laterally during weight-bearing, especially in the heel strike phase of gait [2].

Initially, research emphasized only the role of calf muscles in venous return, largely overlooking the plantar venous pump. This concept, first described in 1890, was initially considered a simple anatomical finding. Lejar's early work identified the superficial venous network in the sole of the foot as the main venous reservoir. It took over a century for this concept to be challenged. Uhl and Gillot's dissection of 400 cadaveric subjects revealed that the true venous reservoir of the foot is deep within the plantar muscles. This new, more physiologic concept of the plantar venous pump involves plantar veins converging into a venous system, initiating an upward venous return with each step [3]. The foot has five venous systems: the superficial dorsal plexus, the superficial plantar veins, the perforating veins, the marginal veins, and the deep plantar veins. The biomechanical influence primarily stems from the plantar and perforating venous structures (Fig. 9.1).

Pathophysiology

Contrary to popular belief, the heart is not the primary pump for the venous system. Venous return from the lower extremities heavily relies on the action of the foot, calf, and thigh muscle pumps, which together manage approximately 80–90% of the venous return during ambulation. The foot pump is believed to prime the calf to initiate this process.

Variations in foot morphology are multifactorial and influenced by hereditary osseous structures of the foot and lower leg, mobility of soft tissues, and ligamentous laxity. Progressive collapsing flatfoot deformity, also known as posterior tibial tendon dysfunction (PTTD), is a common condition in adults that leads to a flattened arch and often results in a painful and less functional foot [4]. In 2007, Criqui et al. conducted a pivotal population study exploring risk factors for chronic venous disease. Their findings revealed that ligamentous laxity, characterized by flat feet and previous hernia surgery, was predictive of the development of severe venous disease in both males and females. There is compelling evidence that an increase of just 5° in dorsiflexion significantly correlates with the progression of venous disease. This also raises the possibility of connective tissue laxity in the onset of venous conditions [5].

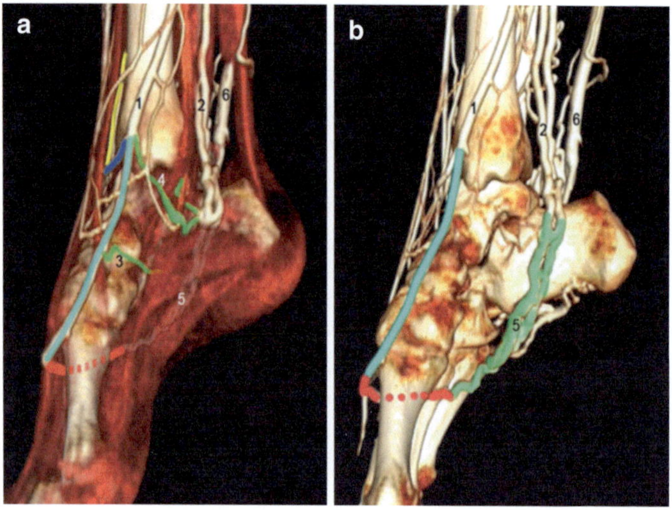

Fig. 9.1 Three-dimensional reconstruction of the roots of the great saphenous vein (GSV), medial perforators, and plantar veins. On the left (**a**), the medial marginal vein is colored in light blue, the anterior tibial veins in yellow, the dorsal communicating vein in dark blue, and the medial perforators in green (3, 4). The perforator vein of the first metatarsal interspace is shown in red. (1): GSV; (2): posterior tibial veins; (3): scaffold perforator; (4): Inframalleolar perforator vein. The lateral plantar veins (5) are seen in transparency through the muscles. (6): SSV, (dilated). On the right (**b**), the tendons and muscles have been removed. The lateral plantar veins (5, in green) and the first metatarsal interspace (in red) are noted. (Courtesy of Uhl and Gillot). Anatomy of the foot venous pump: physiology and influence on chronic venous disease. (SAGE Publications, 2012)

Two particular foot types, those with hypermobility and pes cavus, have been correlated with venous disease. These correlations likely have two separate causes. Hypermobility in the foot is often found in isolation but can also be associated with conditions such as Ehlers-Danlos syndrome and Down syndrome. A hypermobile foot tends to be flatter and has weaker muscle tone than a less mobile foot. Intrinsic foot muscles are generally weaker unless specifically strengthened.

Consequently, there is likely less force generated by the "foot pump," potentially contributing to the progression of venous disease. In pes cavus, more weight is placed on the lateral aspect of the foot, compressing the lateral plantar vein and altering the mechanics of extrinsic musculature. In 2012, Uhl et al. identified a higher incidence of static foot disorders in individuals with chronic venous disease compared to a control group. Specifically, patients with pes cavus exhibited a higher odds ratio compared to those with pes planus [6]. Uhl delved further into the effects of insoles and compared their impact to compression therapy alone and in combination. Their study indicated an improvement in the quality-of-life score and a reduction in symptoms such as pain, swelling, and heaviness in all three groups, albeit with no additional benefit when used in combination [7, 8].

The calf venous pump manages 65% of the venous return in normal individuals [9, 10]. Superficial venous insufficiency is associated with an estimated 25% reduction of the calf ejection fraction [11]. Bilateral reduced calf pump function has been shown to increase the incidence of thrombosis (hazard ratio [HR], 2.0; 95% CI, 1.2–3.4) [12]. In fact, there is a direct correlation between venous morbidity and venous pump function. About 60% of patients with superficial venous insufficiency have an impaired venous return ejection fraction versus 76% of patients with healed wounds and 90% of those with active ulcers [13].

Differential Diagnosis

Both hypermobile flat feet and pes cavus are frequently associated with foot pain, distinct from venous disease, making it essential to consider differential diagnoses. Several common causes of foot and leg pain, which can be mistaken for venous disease, encompass conditions such as tarsal tunnel syndrome, tendonitis involving the posterior tibial tendon, peroneal tendons, Achilles tendon, and plantar fasciitis. A comprehensive assessment is vital to accurately diagnose and treat these conditions alongside venous disease.

Tarsal tunnel syndrome in the foot is analogous to carpal tunnel syndrome in the hand. It occurs when the posterior tibial nerve becomes compressed within the narrow tarsal tunnel on the medial ankle, which features a thick, overlying retinaculum. This compression may coexist with venous disease, as the posterior tibial vein also traverses the tarsal tunnel. Symptoms of tarsal tunnel syndrome include burning, tingling, numbness, or pain on the plantar aspect of the foot. A positive Tinel's sign test, involving tapping the nerve just behind the medial malleolus, leads to pain or tingling in the nerve's distribution, is indicative of this condition. Electrodiagnostic tests (EMG) can also aid in diagnosis. Treatments for tarsal tunnel syndrome include immobilization, corticosteroid injections, anti-inflammatories, physical therapy, and, in some cases, surgical intervention.

Individuals with pes cavus are particularly susceptible to Achilles tendonitis and peroneal tendonitis. Achilles tendonitis can manifest at various points along the Achilles tendon in the posterior lower leg, with tenderness on palpation of the affected portion. Peroneal tendonitis results from overuse of the evertor muscles, given the natural state of the foot's inverted rearfoot position. It typically presents as lateral ankle or foot pain, often accompanied by pain and inflammation at the base of the 5th metatarsal, where the peroneus brevis inserts onto the bone. Plantar flexion and eversion can elicit pain. The management of both conditions involves physical therapy, orthotics, and bracing. Physical therapy focuses on strengthening the peroneal tendons and stretching the Achilles tendon.

Patients with hypermobility are prone to experiencing posterior tibial tendonitis and plantar fasciitis. These conditions can be effectively treated through physical therapy, emphasizing strengthening intrinsic and extrinsic foot muscles, complemented by orthotics, bracing and injections, to provide necessary support and relief.

Diagnostic and Management

Foot Deformities: Pes Planus, Cavus, Varus, and Valgus

To assess foot deformities, ask the patient to stand barefoot. For a more accurate evaluation, have them march in place briefly and then come to a natural standstill. It would be best to examine the resting calcaneal stance position by observing the patient's posterior heels while standing. Imagine drawing a line bisecting the lower leg and another line bisecting the calcaneus (heel bone). In a neutral arch, these lines will be parallel. In the case of pes planus, the alignment will appear in a valgus position, whereas in a pes cavus foot type, it will display a varus alignment, as illustrated in Fig. 9.2.

Foot type can also be radiographically evaluated using weight-bearing X-rays, although this is typically reserved for cases where clinical concerns necessitate ruling out alternative sources of pain.

Foot Hypermobility: Pes Equinus

Two primary tests are employed to assess hypermobility. The first involves an evaluation of ankle joint dorsiflexion, the preferred method in most studies examining the correlation between hypermobility and vascular disease. The patient should be seated with the knee extended, and dorsiflexion of the foot at the ankle joint should be initiated. To minimize compensation through the midfoot joints, the palm of the hand is placed on the plantar midfoot while dorsiflexing the foot until it reaches its maximum range of motion. The angle between the lower leg along the lateral malleolus and the plantar surface of the lateral foot should be measured. Normal values typically fall between 0° (indicating that the foot is perpendicular to the lower leg) and 20°. Dorsiflexion exceeding 20° is indicative of hypermobility, whereas values below 0° suggest limited dorsiflexion or equinus. Another method for assessing hypermobility, typically employed

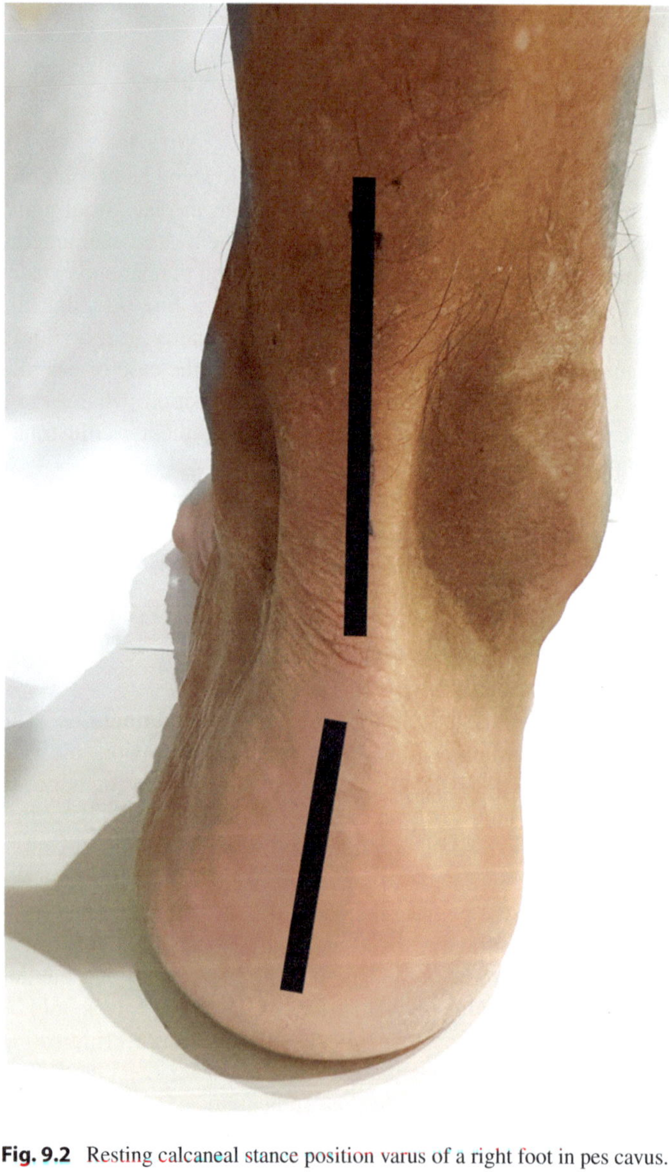

Fig. 9.2 Resting calcaneal stance position varus of a right foot in pes cavus. There is excessive pressure on the lateral aspect of the foot (right side in this picture)

in biomechanics, involves holding the heads of the lesser metatarsals in one hand and the head of the first metatarsal in the other while the patient is in a relaxed seated position. Approximately 5 mm of dorsal and 5 mm of plantar translation is considered within the normal range. Any values exceeding this range are classified as hypermobile (Fig. 9.3).

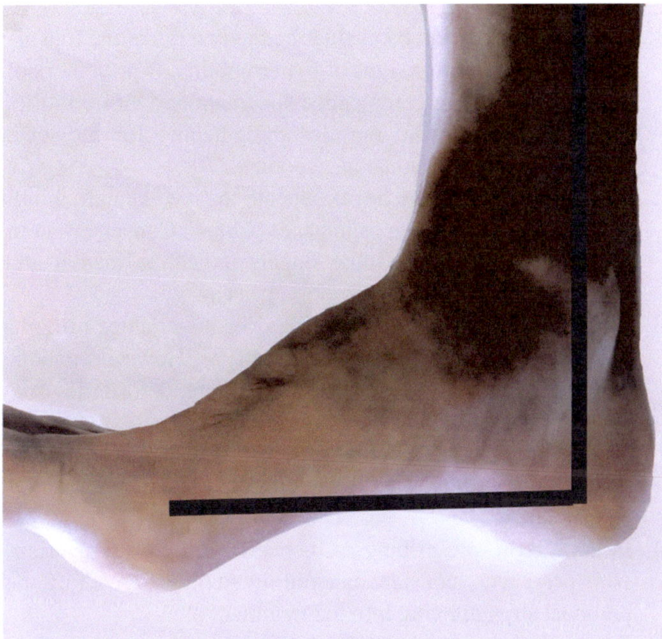

Fig. 9.3 Normal dorsiflexion of approximately 0°. The knee is straight, and a line along the lateral malleolus is connected to a line on the weight-bearing surface of the foot

MGH Additional Tips and Tricks

Saggini et al. explored the effects of arch-specific insoles. They found that their usage enhanced venous emptying capacity, which they attributed to an improvement in the activation of the plantar vein complex. At MGH, we usually recommend the following:

1. Begin the assessment by evaluating the first ray of the foot and ankle dorsiflexion for signs of hypermobility. If present, podiatry evaluation is recommended for treatment with orthotics. Intrinsic and extrinsic muscle strengthening for the lower extremities should also be incorporated.
2. If you cannot slide one finger beneath the medial arch, it indicates a flatter foot, often called "pes planus." Conversely, comfortably fitting two or more fingers under the medial arch indicates a higher arch, known as "pes cavus."
3. Treatment may be initiated with over-the-counter orthotics tailored to the patient's specific foot type. However, patients with very high arches or additional foot deformities may require custom-molded orthotics. In our practice, this is a critical adjuvant or alternative to compression for patients unable or unwilling to wear stockings to manage their venous insufficiency.
4. In addition to prescribing arch-specific orthotics for patients with pes cavus, consider integrating Achilles stretching and peroneal strengthening into the treatment plan.
5. Be mindful that orthotics often necessitate larger shoe sizes, which can pose challenges for patients with lower extremity edema. Consider recommending extra-width and extra-depth shoes when indicated.
6. Prescribe exercises that stimulate the intrinsic muscles of the foot and promote plantar venous pump function, especially in cases of if sedentary lifestyle, prolonged sitting, or prolonged standing.

Summary

The discovery that the true venous reservoir is located deep within the plantar muscles rather than superficially has significant implications for the treatment and management of venous insufficiency and static foot disorders. It highlights the need for a more comprehensive approach to studying and treating venous pathology, considering the complex interplay of various anatomical and physiological factors.

Evaluating foot type and hypermobility is a crucial aspect of the physical examination for vascular disease. Pes cavus and excessive ankle joint dorsiflexion are correlated with superficial venous insufficiency. Orthotics have shown promise in alleviating symptoms and should be integrated into the treatment regimen, tailored to the patient's arch type.

References

1. Ludbrook J. The musculovenous pumps of the human lower limb. Am Heart J. 1966;71(5):635–41. https://doi.org/10.1016/0002-8703(66)90313-9. PMID: 5935855.
2. Binns M, Pho RW. Anatomy of the 'venous foot pump'. Injury. 1988;19(6):443–5. https://doi.org/10.1016/0020-1383(88)90144-1. PMID: 3267655.
3. Uhl J-F, Gillot C. Anatomy of the foot venous pump: physiology and influence on chronic venous disease. Phlebology. 2012;27:219–30.
4. Myerson MS, Thordarson DB, Johnson JE, Hintermann B, Sangeorzan BJ, Deland JT, Schon LC, Ellis SJ, de Cesar NC. Classification and nomenclature: progressive collapsing foot deformity. Foot Ankle Int. 2020;41(10):1271–6. https://doi.org/10.1177/1071100720950722. Epub 2020 Aug 28. PMID: 32856474.
5. Kim TI, Forbang NI, Criqui MH, Allison MA. Association of foot and ankle characteristics with progression of venous disease. Vasc Med. 2015;20(2):105–11. https://doi.org/10.1177/1358863X14568443. PMID: 25832598.
6. Uhl JF, Chahim M, Allaert FA. Static foot disorders: a major risk factor for chronic venous disease? Phlebology. 2012;27(1):13–8. https://doi.org/10.1258/phleb.2011.010060. Epub 2011 Jul 4. PMID: 21727156.
7. Uhl JF, Chahim M, Allaert FA. Compression versus inner sole for venous patients with foot static disorders: a prospective trial comparing symp-

toms and quality of life. Phlebology. 2015;30(1):32–8. https://doi.org/10.1177/0268355513505508. Epub 2013 Sep 27. PMID: 24077127.

8. Saggini R, Bellomo RG, Iodice P, Lessiani G. Venous insufficiency and foot dysmorphism: effectiveness of visco-elastic rehabilitation systems on veno-muscle system of the foot and of the calf. Int J Immunopathol Pharmacol. 2009;22(3 Suppl):1–8. https://doi.org/10.1177/03946320090220S301. PMID: 19887035.
9. Niccolini G, Manuello A, Capone A, Marongiu G, Dell'Osa Antonio H, Fois A, Velluzzi F, Concu A. Possible assessment of calf venous pump efficiency by computational fluid dynamics approach. Front Physiol. 2020;11. https://doi.org/10.3389/fphys.2020.01003.
10. Williams KJ, et al. The calf muscle pump revisited. J Vasc Surg Venous Lymphat Disord. 2014;2(3):329–34.
11. Kan YM, Delis KT. Hemodynamic effects of supervised calf muscle exercise in patients with venous leg ulceration: a prospective controlled study. Arch Surg. 2001;136(12):1364–9. https://doi.org/10.1001/archsurg.136.12.1364.
12. Houghton DE, Ashrani A, Liedl D, Mehta RA, Hodge DO, Rooke T, Wennberg P, Wysokinski W, McBane R. Reduced calf muscle pump function is a risk factor for venous thromboembolism: a population-based cohort study. Blood. 2021;137(23):3284–90. https://doi.org/10.1182/blood.2020010231.
13. Araki CT, Back TL, Padberg FT, et al. The significance of calf muscle pump function in venous ulceration. J Vasc Surg. 1994;20:872–9.

Lymphedema as a Differential Diagnosis of the Swollen Limb

10

Lynn Gray-Meltzer, Cheryl L. Brunelle,
Carlos Echevarria,
and Jonathan Winograd

Cardiac, hepatic, and renal conditions, among other systemic problems, can manifest as lower limb edema. Chronic venous insufficiency (CVI) is the most common singular cause of lower extremity edema in individuals over 50 years old [1], but additional differential diagnoses include skin conditions such as cel-

L. Gray-Meltzer · C. L. Brunelle (✉)
Department of Physical and Occupational Therapy,
Massachusetts General Hospital, Boston, MA, USA
e-mail: lfgray@mgb.org; lgray-meltzer@mghihp.edu; cbrunelle@mgh.harvard.edu

C. Echevarria
Division of Vascular and Endovascular Surgery, Department of Surgery,
Massachusetts General Hospital/Harvard Venous & Lymphatic Medicine Alumni, Boston, MA, USA

Division of Vascular Medicine and Endovenous Interventions,
Veins & Vascular Centers of Excellence, Phoenix, AZ, USA
e-mail: carlos.echevarria@vascular.md

J. Winograd
Plastic and Reconstructive Surgery, Massachusetts General Hospital
Lymphedema Center of Excellence, Boston, MA, USA
e-mail: jwinograd@mgh.harvard.edu

C. Echevarria et al. (eds.), *The Massachusetts General Hospital Protocols and Procedures for Venous Disease*,
https://doi.org/10.1007/978-3-032-05708-2_10

lulitis, muscle swelling caused by trauma, bony changes or muscular impairments that affect a limb's muscle pump functions, arterial swelling after revascularization, and lymphatic disease. As previous chapters have extensively discussed CVI, this chapter will cover in detail an often overlooked and misunderstood differential diagnosis for lower limb swelling: lymphedema.

Lymphedema

Up to ten million Americans and 250 million people worldwide suffer from lymphatic diseases [2]. This is more than human immunodeficiency virus and Parkinson's disease combined, yet lymphedema remains an underrecognized, poorly understood, and underfunded condition [1, 3, 4]. Lower extremity swelling is frequently labeled lymphedema in the absence of defining etiology, which is frequently a mixture of local and systemic pathologies. These chronic changes negatively impact physical and mental health and significantly worsen quality of life (QOL) due to discomfort, disfigurement, and decreased activity [1, 3, 5–8].

Lymphedema is a chronic, dynamic, and progressive disease in which protein-rich fluid accumulates in the interstitial space. Non-valved superficial dermal lymphatics drain into subdermal channels in the superficial venous system. Lymph then flows unidirectionally into deeper, valved, smooth-muscle-lined trunks in the epifascial and subfascial systems and eventually to lymph nodes and the vena cava via the subclavian veins [9, 10]

Primary lymphedema can result from a congenital defect or absence of lymphatic vessels, and it is classified by age group: congenital (0–1 year), praecox (ages 2–35 years), and lymphedema tarda (after 35 years old) [11]. Secondary lymphedema is due to damage or overflow of the lymphatic vessels or nodes, affecting the normal forward flow of the lymphatic system.

Staging of Lymphedema: The International Society of Lymphedema staging system, outlined in Table 10.1, is most used for assessment of the condition

Decreased ability to absorb excess water and protein from the interstitium reduces transport capacity, creating an insufficiency

Table 10.1 International society of lymphology lymphedema staging system [12]

International society of lymphedema stage	Characteristics of stage
0	Latent or subclinical lymphedema, with abnormal lymph transport, subtle alterations in tissue fluid/composition, and changes in subjective symptoms.
1	Early protein-rich fluid accumulation, pitting edema may occur, improves with limb elevation.
2	Pitting is evident, edema does not resolve with elevation alone. Pitting will decrease in later stage 2 with tissue changes including subcutaneous fat and fibrosis.
3	Fibroadipose deposition and skin changes are evident, pitting becomes absent.

in the lymphatic system. Over time, extravascular protein stimulates proliferation of fibroblasts, potentially causing a limb to become fibrotic, non-pitting, and "woody" in later stages. Accumulated proteins and fluid stasis provide an opportunistic environment for microbial growth, while lymphatic dysfunction decreases local immune responses, predisposing these patients to recurrent infection (cellulitis) [13, 14]. This staging system has limitations, as it does not specify lymphatic changes during each stage or take into consideration the patient experience, such as aching, tightness, heaviness, or changes in limb function [15]. It does, however, offer some guidance on the potential clinical or surgical interventions that could benefit these patients.

Etiologies of Swelling and Differential Diagnosis

Given the high prevalence of mixed etiology in lower extremity swelling, precise differential diagnosis is key to optimizing the patient plan of care and facilitating a good patient outcome. In order to help guide the clinician, common causes of mixed etiology swelling, related clinical presentation, and diagnostic testing are outlined in Table 10.2.

Table 10.2 Etiology, clinical presentation, and key diagnostic tests for swelling of the lower extremity

Etiology of bilateral edema	Clinical presentation/ signs and symptoms	Key auxiliary diagnostic testing
Systemic		
Cardiac (heart failure)	Pitting edema in legs, ankles, or feet [16] Dyspnea on exertion, orthopnea [16] Irregular rhythm, chest pain, or pressure [16]	Chest x-ray [16] Electrocardiogram (ECG) B-type natriuretic peptide [16] Echocardiography [16] Graded exercise stress test [17, 18] Multiple-gated acquisition (MUGA) scanning [19]
Renal disease [20]	Edema of lower limbs unrelated to time of the day Periorbital puffiness, especially in the morning Fatigue Decreased appetite Muscle cramping at night	Urinalysis ➔ urinary protein/creatinine ratio >200 mg/g (proteinuria), urinary albumin/creatinine ratio >30 mg/g Glomerular Filtration Rate (GFR) Sodium, potassium [21, 22] Hemoglobin A1C [21] Doppler ultrasonography [20, 23]
Hepatic disease [24]	Pitting edema in the legs, ankles, or feet Clubbing, nail changes Jaundice of the skin and eyes Telangiectasias, abdominal wall vascular collaterals (caput medusae) [24] Ascites Asterixis and encephalopathy	Liver panel Complete blood count (CBC) with platelets and prothrombin time [24] Ultrasonography CT and MRI Sodium levels (hyponatremia is assoc. with poor prognosis of end-stage liver disease)

(continued)

Table 10.2 (continued)

Venous insufficiency/ stasis [25]	Leg discomfort, often described as heaviness or aching after prolonged standing, relieved by elevation of the leg Telangiectasis or reticular veins, superficial thrombophlebitis (painful, indurated, inflamed areas along the varicose veins) Edema (begins in the perimalleolar region and ascends up the leg with dependent fluid accumulation) Skin changes and lesions: hemosiderin changes (red or brown discoloration), eczema, lipodermatosclerosis, and venous ulceration [25]	Venous duplex ultrasound Computed tomography and magnetic resonance venography Contrast venography [25]
Lymphatic		
Primary lymphedema: Congenital (Milroy) Praecox (Meige) Tarda [26–28]	Childhood onset is most common Almost exclusively affects lower extremities May present unilaterally Non-pitting edema, skin changes: peau d'orange, pinkish-red discoloration, dermatitis, eczema, etc. [29] Positive Stemmer sign [30] Family history	X-rays to look for bone abnormalities of phleboliths (as venous malformation can be comorbid) [29] Venous duplex ultrasound [29] Lymphoscintigraphy
Secondary lymphedema:		

(continued)

Table 10.2 (continued)

Filariasis	Travel to area endemic to filariasis: Africa: Sub-Saharan Africa, Egypt Asia: Southeast Asia, the Indian subcontinent Pacific: Some southwestern Pacific Islands Americas: Northeastern coast of Brazil, Guayana, and Hispaniola (Dominican Republic, Haiti) Red skin patches, whole leg swelling Fever, shivering, myalgias Elephantiasis, hydrocele [31]	Blood smear with microscopic examination Alere Filariasis Test Strip (FTS) [32]
Metastatic malignant disease	Sudden onset and rapidly worsening swelling, especially with oncology history	Abdominal/pelvic CT or MRI of leg as appropriate to check for mass and vessel obstruction
Cancer treatments	Lower extremity lymphedema can be uni- or bilateral post PLND Gradual onset, non-tender, usually in distal extremity (including foot), progressing proximally Pitting edema with indentations around borders of socks/shoes, thickened skin, peau d'orange, progressing to non-pitting edema in later stages Positive Stemmer sign Erythema Sometimes immobile, dense scars or radiation fibrosis [1, 12, 33]	Rule out cancer recurrence Rule out infection Ultrasonography Lymphoscintigraphy Magnetic resonance lymphangiography (MRL) (function of lymphatics, characteristics of limb, visualization of nodal basin) [33] Indocyanine green (ICG) lymphangiography (real-time visualization of lymphatic flow) [33] Prospective surveillance using relative volume change, ideally with preoperative baseline [34–37] or utilize bioimpedance spectroscopy [38, 39]

(continued)

Table 10.2 (continued)

Other		
Lipedema [40]	Subcutaneous fat depositions at buttocks and thighs out of proportion to the upper body Mild edema initially, usually spares feet Achy pain and tenderness of the skin of the lower extremities with any pressure [9, 41]	MRI (looking for abnormally high fat deposition) [41] Lymphoscintigraphy (would expect normal findings compared to classic lymphedema) [42]
Etiology of Unilateral edema	**Clinical presentation/ signs and symptoms**	**Key diagnostic tests**
Vascular or orthopedic		
Vascular insufficiency due to previous trauma or surgery that was unilateral [25]	Dense superficial and deep scar tissue Reduced fascia and joint mobility Lesions on the skin, red or brown discolorations Scaling and crust [25]	Tests for heart, kidney, and liver function, especially if the swelling could be truly bilateral asymmetrical vs unilateral, and there is not actually an uninvolved limb Duplex ultrasound (DUS) [1] If additional imaging of the abdomen or pelvis is necessary after DUS, contrast-enhanced venous phase computed tomography (CT) or magnetic resonance venous (MRV) imaging [1] Venography with intravascular ultrasound (IVUS) [1]
Deep vein thrombosis (DVT)	Swollen, or tender limb, sometimes with focal erythema, rapid onset Scores ≥2 on Wells criteria [43–45] Among major lower limb surgeries, advanced age, female gender, and TKR most increase risk for DVT [29]	DUS [1] (consider highest venous thromboembolism risk intraoperative-3 months post-op after major orthopedic surgery) [46] Supine Doppler

(continued)

Table 10.2 (continued)

Orthopedic surgery or injury (ex. joint replacement, sprain/strain)	Edema usually mostly at and below the knee Mild swelling can be normal up to 6 months after TKR, peak swelling occurs between day 1 and 90 post op [47] and presents in at least 90.7% of patients [48] Decreased activity (increased risk for DVT with lack of early mobilization postoperatively)	Rule out DVT (consider highest venous thromboembolism risk intraoperative-3 months post op after major orthopedic surgery [46] Rule out infection X-ray MRI
Lymphatic		
Secondary lymphedema (secondary to surgery, lymph node removal, scar tissue, and nodal radiation of unilateral nature)	Gradual onset, progressive if untreated Foot and digit involvement common Peak lower extremity lymphedema incidence 6–12 months post-op, then tapers over 2+ years [3] Similar characteristics to bilateral lower extremity lymphedema, but unilateral Small transitions in limb volume change are common, but rapidly worsening is abnormal [10]	Ultrasonography to rule out DVT as indicated Lymphoscintigraphy Indocyanine green lymphography NB: Oncology history + acutely swollen limb should raise concern for cellulitis, DVT, radiotherapy-induced venous stenosis (RIVS)—rare but mimic of DVT [49] Prospective surveillance using relative volume change [34–37] or bioimpedance spectroscopy
Primary lymphedema	Usually bilateral, but can be unilateral if there is a unilateral defect in the structure [26]	Lymphoscintigraphy Bioimpedance spectroscopy [26]

Medication-Induced Edema

Edema can be a side effect of several medications. All current or recently discontinued medications should be reconciled, including recent changes and self-dosing. Cardiac medications such as renin-angiotensin-aldosterone system inhibitors (RAASi), calcium channel blockers (CCB), beta blockers (BB), hydralazine, and others may raise suspicion for edema due to cardiac disease, even in the absence of a patient's recollection of a formal diagnosis. However, most importantly is recognizing that some of these medications may cause edema per se [50]. The pathophysiology of drug-induced edema is multifactorial, and although multiple pathways have been identified, this is our attempt to categorize medication-induced edema by mechanism of action:

Vasodilation

Vasodilation of precapillary arterioles can increase capillary hydrostatic pressure, leading to fluid extravasation into the interstitial space. The following medications increase risk of limb swelling related to vasodilation:

Antihypertensives	CCB, Minoxidil, Hydralazine
Antiparkinsonian drugs	Pramipexole, levodopa, amantadine
Antidepressants 5-HT2 antagonists	Olanzapine, mirtazapine, trazodone, quetiapine, clozapine, risperidone, triptilines, citalopram, tramadol, fluoxetine, cyclobenzaprine, aripiprazole
Gabapentinoids	Gabapentin, pregabalin, baclofen
Endothelin receptor antagonists	Bosentan for pulmonary vasoconstriction

The occurrence of edema due to CCB is more common with dihydropyridine medications, such as amlodipine and nifedipine, compared to non-dihydropyridine CCBs like verapamil and diltiazem. As people age, the balance between transcapillary flow and its compensatory mechanisms becomes more fragile. Notably, about 25% of individuals with a mean age of 55 years on CCB have such complications within the first year of treatment [51]. Depending on the clinical context, the clinician may consider dose reduction, CCB cessation, switching to non-dihydropyridine CCBs, or a different blood pressure medication. Alternatively, an elegant strategy of adding an RAAS inhibitor may reduce CCB-induced edema by decreasing postcapillary pressure, causing vasodilation and thereby reducing fluid extravasation [52].

Drug-Induced Sodium/Water Retention

The mechanism of action that causes salt and water retention associated with medication is also called renal-induced edema. Some medications that may induce sodium and water retention are listed below:

Hormones or hormonal inhibitors	Danazol, testosterone, progestin, tamoxifen, aromatase inhibitors
Corticosteroids	Prednisone, hydrocortisone
Analgesic and anti-inflammatories	NSAIDs, opioids
Antihypertensives	Alpha blockers, minoxidil, hydralazine

Depending on the medication, the effect may be caused by sodium retention through increased proximal tubular reabsorption, mineralocorticoid effect, prostaglandin inhibition of natriuresis and aquaresis, or RAAS stimulation.

Transcapillary Permeability

Transcapillary permeability is a common condition induced by anticancer drugs called Capillary Leak Syndrome (CLS). Examples of anticancer drugs that frequently cause CLS are listed here:

Cytokines	Interleukin-2, granulocyte colony-stimulating factor
Antineoplastic agents	Gemcitabine and clofarabine, imatinib and dasatinib

Some of these medications may interfere with the signaling pathways involved in endothelial permeability. Kinase inhibitors are known to cause periorbital and/or extremity edema in 74%–84% of imatinib-treated patients) [53].

Impaired Lymphatic Flow

Some drugs cause reduced lymphatic flow due to impairment of lymphatic peristalsis. Also, some of these drugs interfere with vascular endothelial growth factors (VEGFs) that promote lymphangiogenesis. Examples of drugs that may interfere with VEGFs are listed here:

Antiestrogens	Tamoxifen
Taxanes	Paclitaxel [39] and docetaxel [40]
mTOR inhibitors	Everolimus, sirolimus [51]
PI3K/AKT inhibitors [50]	Alpelisib, idelalisib

It has been our experience at MGH that 6.8%–9.2% of a cohort of 160 patients on PI3K, Mtor, or CDK4/6 inhibitor for metastatic breast cancer experienced new onset or worsened preexisting upper extremity edema in the limb at risk for lymphedema after breast cancer treatment [54]. The risk of limb lymphedema imparted by such targeted therapies requires further investigation but should be considered by the clinician when discussing potential side effects.

Cancer-Specific Risk Factors for Lower Limb Lymphedema

Aside from CVI progressively affecting the lymphatic system (phlebolymphedema), cancer treatments, specifically lymph node removal and regional nodal irradiation, are the most common cause of secondary lymphedema in Western countries [7, 12]. Treatment of gynecologic and prostatic malignancies results in the highest incidence of secondary lower extremity lymphedema, as summarized in Table 10.3.

Table 10.3 Cancer-related lymphedema of the lower extremity: incidence and study characteristics

Cancer type	Study (*N*)	Incidence	Diagnostic criteria for lymphedema	Follow-up time
Endometrial	Salani et al. 2014 [55] (482)	35% of cohort reported any swelling 22.3% of cohort reported formal diagnosis	Self-report	3+ years post diagnosis (cross-sectional)
	Carlson et al. 2020 [10] (1054)	34%	Limb volume change ≥10% from pre-operative baseline	24 months
Cervical	Carlson et al. 2020 [10] (1054)	35%	Limb volume change ≥10% from pre-operative baseline	24 months
Vulvar	Carlson et al. 2020 [10] (1054)	43%	Limb volume change ≥10% from pre-operative baseline	24 months
Prostate cancer: RP + RNI	Clinckaert et al. 2022 [15] (99–3675, total 9223)	0%–9%	Self-report, undefined	Varied: 28 days to >15 years, or not reported
Prostate cancer: RP + PLND	Raskin et al. 2019 [56] (139)	20.8%	"Standardized manner," undefined	Not reported
	Clinckaert et al. 2022 [15] (99–3675, total 9223)	0%–14%	Self-report, undefined	Varied: 28 days to >15 years, or not reported
Prostate cancer: RP + PLND + RNI	Clinckaert et al. 2022 [15] (99–3675, total 9223)	18%–29%	Self-report, undefined	Varied: 28 days to >15 years, or not reported

(continued)

Table 10.3 (continued)

Cancer type	Study (*N*)	Incidence	Diagnostic criteria for lymphedema	Follow-up time
Melanoma	Woon et al. 2023 [57] (81)	51% post inguinal LND; 62% post ilioinguinal LND	Physical examination including: Stemmer's sign, pitting, skin changes, volumetric difference in limbs	15 months
	Hyngstrom et al. 2013 [58] (90)	23% post inguinofemoral surgery	Limb volume measured with perometer at pre-operative baseline and 6 and 12 months post op	12 months

Abbreviations: *RP* radical prostatectomy, *RNI* regional nodal irradiation, *LND* lymph node dissection, *PLND* pelvic lymph node dissection

In a meta-analysis of 3401 patients treated for cervical cancer, the main risk factors identified for lower extremity lymphedema after gynecologic cancer treatment were: body mass index (BMI) (OR = 1.37, 95% CI: 1.10–1.71, $P = 0.005$), age (OR = 1.68, 95% CI: 1.07–2.64, $P = 0.02$), International Federation of Gynecology and Obstetrics (FIGO) stage (OR = 1.50, 95% CI: 1.24–1.82, $P < 0.001$), radiotherapy (OR = 2.87, 95% CI: 1.71–4.82, $P < 0.001$), lymph node (LN) dissection (OR = 3.24, 95% CI: 1.44–7.31, $P = 0.005$), and the number of LNs dissected (OR = 2.34, 95% CI: 1.80–3.05, $P < 0.001$) [59]. Carlson et al. found an increased risk of lower extremity lymphedema after endometrial cancer with removal of >8 LN [8, 10]. Regional nodal irradiation has been found to be an independent risk factor for lower extremity lymphedema (OR 3.81, 95% CI 1.67–8.69) [14, 60]. Similar correlations have been found in other studies, regardless of the cancer type.

Patient Reported Symptoms

A complete patient history facilitates accurate, efficient, and cost-effective diagnostic testing and management [1]. As a result, several symptom screening tools have been developed to aid diagnosis of disease, symptom monitoring, and capture the patient experience; these are called *Patient Reported Outcome Measures* (PROMs), some of which are presented below (Table 10.4).

Table 10.4 Patient-reported outcome measures for lower extremity lymphedema

PROMs	Description
Lower Extremity Lymphedema (LEL) Screening Questionnaire	Self-report screener, developed to detect LEL in both normal-weight and obese patients Cut score of 5 for detecting LEL; depending on BMI <30 kg/m^2 or BMI ≥30 kg/m^2 Sensitivity and Specificity were 94.8%–95.5% and 76.5%–86.5% respectively [61, 62]
Lymphedema Symptom Intensity and Distress Survey-Lower Limb (LSIDS-L)	Brief self-report tool for monitoring symptoms over time Not for detection and screening [3] Focused on understanding impact and burden [63]
Lymphedema Life Impact Scale (LLIS) [64–66]	Self-report, lymphedema-specific tool, 18 questions regarding symptoms over the previous week, addressing three subscales: physical, psychosocial, and functional Accuracy 97%, Sensitivity 100%, and Specificity 84.8% at a cutoff of C 5.88 overall percent impairment score (higher scores indicate worse disability) [66]
Gynecological Cancer Lymphedema Questionnaire (GCLQ) [3]	Self-report, 20 questions assessing 20 symptoms associated with LEL Modification of the validated Lymphedema Breast Cancer Q Appropriate for screening or intervention in a clinical setting Cut score of ≥4 from baseline is significantly associated with LEL [3]
Lymphedema of the Limbs—Quality of Life (LYMQOL LEG) [67]	Self-report, 27 item (leg-version) 4 domains: function, body image/appearance, symptoms, mood Reliability intra-class-correlation coefficient 0.78–0.90 (leg-version), internal consistency Cronbach's alpha values 0.87–0.97 (leg-version)

Abbreviation: *LEL* lower extremity lymphedema

Clinical Exam

Lymphedema diagnosis should integrate data from patient-reported symptoms, clinical examination, and measurement of limb volume or extracellular fluid [5, 15]

Skin Inspection and Palpation assess tissue texture, pitting, wounds, and overall appearance. The pitting test is considered an indicator of excess free fluid that has accumulated in the interstitial tissue space [68]. *Pitting edema measurement* should be standardized with 30 s moderate pressure applied to the body surface [69, 70], then released and graded: **1+** Barely detectable impression when finger pressed into skin; **2+** Slight indentation, 15 s to rebound; **3+** Deeper indentation, 30 s to rebound; **4+** >30 s to rebound [71].

Stemmer Sign associates the inability to pinch the skin over the proximal second toe with the existence of abnormal dermal backflow in lower extremity lymphedema [72, 73]. A positive Stemmer sign (*inability* to pinch the skin) is a sensitive predictor of lymphedema, but without a strong clinical correlation, its specificity is poor (sensitivity 92%, specificity 57%) [74]. Adjunct testing may be considered.

Screen for conditions that may require immediate attention first. Evaluate resting vitals, skin integrity check, venous and arterial flow (pedal pulses, jugular venous distention, Buerger's test, Ankle Brachial Index), and lung auscultation to rule out pulmonary edema or pleural effusions. Suspicion of thrombosis-induced edema would be a more imminent event but, when in doubt, apply the Wells criteria to rule out DVT rather than relying on the physical exam alone (the Wells criteria has 100% sensitivity, 100% negative predictive value, and 90% accuracy vs. Homan's sign positive predictive value of 50% [75]).

Objective Measurement of Edema

Objective measurement of limb volume or fluid status is imperative to both monitor for changes with treatment of edema or monitor for development of secondary lymphedema. There are several valid and reliable options for measurement, including limb volume methods (tape measure, optoelectronic volumeter, or 3D camera) or measures of tissue fluid status (bioimpedance spectroscopy or tissue dielectric constant). Several methods are briefly summarized here.

Tape Measure: Girth measures are completed with a flexible tape measure and converted to volume using the truncated cone formula and commercially available software. Measurement recommendations include: bony landmark visualization and tape measurements of circumference every 4 or 10 cm on the limb with a flexible measuring tape. It is recommended to compare to the contralateral side when normal. In case of malignancy, obtain preoperative baseline measurements for future comparison [10, 76] For unilateral edema, leg volumes at baseline and follow-up should be converted to a Relative Volume Change (RVC) (percent from preoperative baseline) whenever possible using the following formula:

$$\text{RVC} = \left[\frac{A_2 U_1}{U_2 A_1} - 1\right] \times 100\%$$

where: A: affected limb volume, U: unaffected limb volume, 2: follow-up, and 1: pre-op baseline [77].

For bilateral edema, leg volumes should be compared to baseline values and data integrated with clinical exam and symptom report. When utilizing girth measures, absolute differences in circumference (2 cm) or volume (200 mL) should not be used in isolation but as corroboration of a clinical diagnosis of lymphedema [34]. This is because legs are asymmetrical at the preoperative baseline, and without incorporation of this asymmetry, misdiagnosis is significant. In these cases, history, clinical exam and symptomatology should be heavily weighted.

Optoelectronic Limb Volumetry/Perometer (Fig. 10.1) is a valid, reliable, rapid, highly reproducible method to assess limb volume measurements [78–82]. The limb is flanked by a series of LED lights and opposing photosensors that scan the diameter of the upper or lower extremities in a geometrical fashion. Challenges include significant upfront cost and space requirements [76]

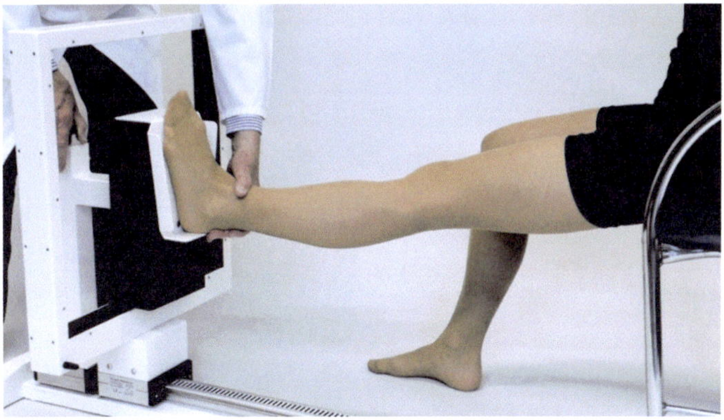

Fig. 10.1 Lower extremity optoelectronic limb volumeter. Lower extremity volume measurement via perometry. (Note: Picture courtesy of Pero-System Messgeraete GmbH, Wuppertal, Germany)

Bio-impedance Spectroscopy (BIS) (Fig. 10.2), which evaluates the resistance of alternating electrical current of the extracellular and intracellular space, may be used to characterize excess extracellular fluid [15]. It may be used for bilateral lower extremity lymphedema (where there is not an unaffected limb for volume comparison), measurements are rapid and reproducible. However, there are upfront and monthly costs associated with the device, it requires space, and during later stages in which the tissue is fat-dominant, this method may not identify lymphedema [3, 83–87]

3D Camera: A 3D camera attached to an iPad with associated software to capture limb volume (Fig. 10.3) highly correlates with perometry and is a rapid and portable method of capturing limb volume. Volumes may be entered into the RVC equation to capture changes from preoperative baselines. There are upfront and monthly costs associated with this device.

Tissue Dielectric Constant measurement provides a quantitative index of skin water content associated with lymphedema. An integrated probe with a built-in pressure sensor displays percent tissue water content [88]. The device (either the LymphScanner or

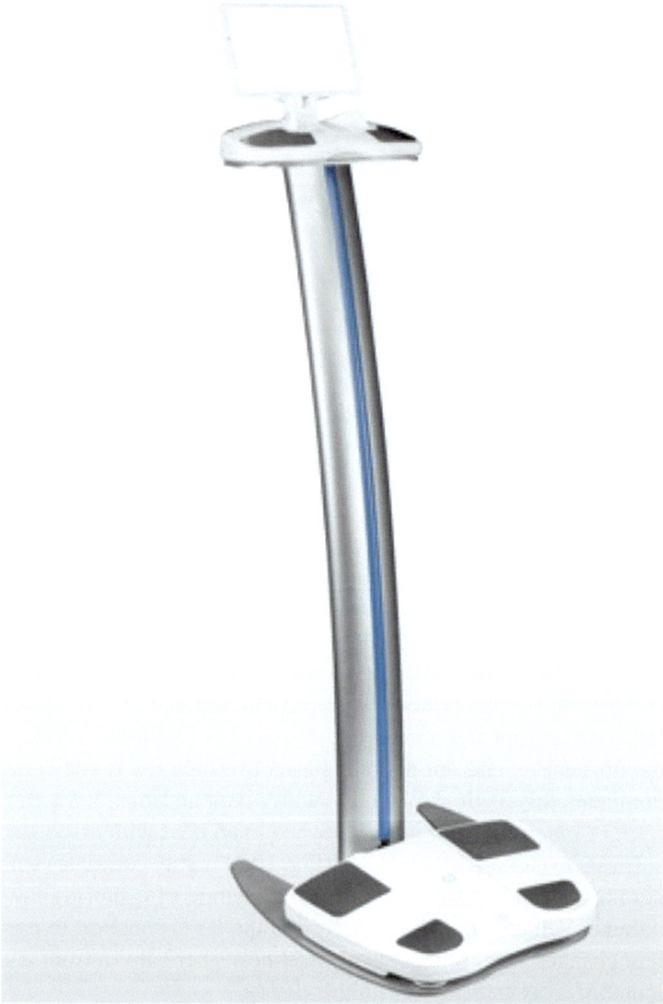

Fig. 10.2 Bioelectrical impedance spectroscopy (BIS) SOZO® Digital Health Platform. Bioimpedence spectroscopy uses bioimpedance measurements to assess fluid levels and tissue composition. (*Note:* Picture courtesy of ImpediMed Limited, Pinkenba, QLD 4008, Australia)

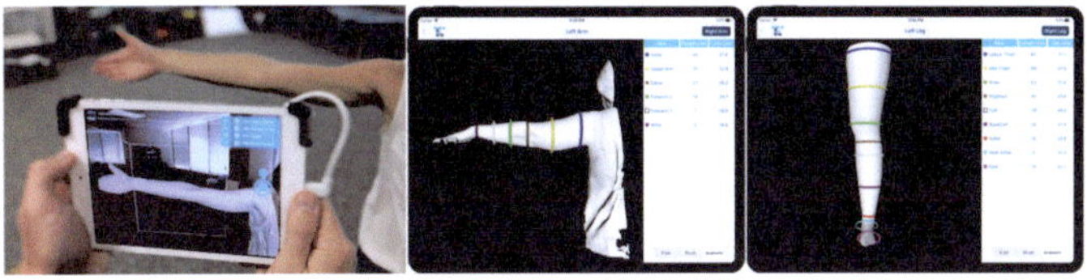

Fig. 10.3 3D camera, iPad, and software imaging to capture lower extremity volume. Capturing limb size measurements via 3D camera scanning with an iPad is promising for clinical utility due to its portability and speed compared to circumferential measurements done with tape. (Note: Picture courtesy of LymphaTech, Inc., Atlanta, GA)

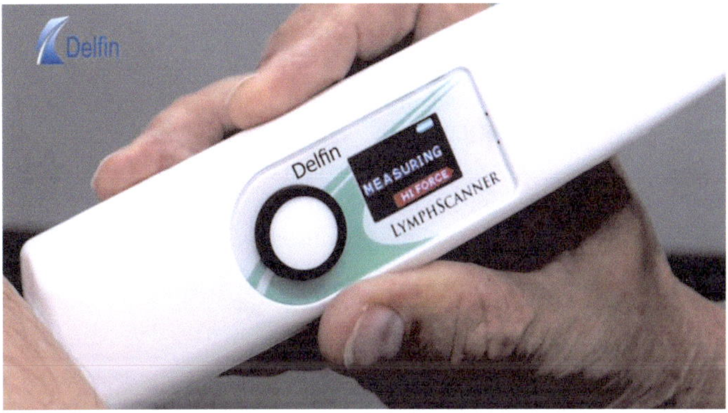

Fig. 10.4 MoistureMeterD Compact. A hand-held tool for measuring tissue dielectric constant to quantify skin water content. (*Note*: Picture courtesy of Delfin Technologies Ltd., Kuopio, Finland)

MoistureMeter D Compact) (Fig. 10.4) is a portable, valid, and reliable method of evaluation of limb edema and has the additional benefit of being able to measure trunk and breast edema. There are upfront costs associated with this device.

An Important Differential Diagnosis

Lipedema

Lipedema, sometimes confused with lymphedema, affects approximately 11% of females [40]

Lipedema is a highly underdiagnosed, chronic, congenital condition, often confused with standard obesity and erroneously diagnosed as lymphedema. However, unlike lymphedema, it is not characterized by a dysfunctional lymphatic system. Lipedema is a painful condition characterized by symmetrical, abnormal deposition of adipose tissue in the limbs, which spares the hands and feet. It also affects the lower trunk in some patients. It almost exclusively appears in females and most often presents around times of drastic hormonal changes, such as puberty and menopause [40]. Classification of lipedema by staging and type is outlined in Table 10.5. It should be noted that a fourth stage of lipedema has been suggested, consisting of lipedema with lymphedema. Lipedema is a treatable condition, with several novel con-

Table 10.5 Lipedema staging and type classifications [89, 90]

Lipedema stage	Stage characterized by
1	Skin has a smooth texture with a subdermal pebble-like feel due to underlying loose connective tissue fibrosis.
2	Skin dimpling due to progressed fibrotic changes and excess tissue. Palpable nodules may be more numerous and larger.
3	Increased lipedema tissue, more fibrotic in texture, with numerous large subdermal nodules and overhanging lobules of tissue
Lipedema type	**Anatomical location**
1	Buttocks, pelvis, and hips only
2	Buttocks to knees
3	Buttocks to ankles
4	Arms only
5	Lower leg only

sensus documents available to guide the clinician [89, 91, 92]. Unfortunately, since knowledge of this condition is evolving among healthcare providers, it is underrecognized, and many patients go without treatment well into adulthood.

Diagnosis and Management of Lymphedema

As a designated Center of Excellence by the Lymphatic Education and Research Network (LERN), the MGH Lymphatic Program follows the LERN protocol for patient management (see Fig. 10.5). This involves a screening duplex ultrasound combined with clinical examination to sort lipedema, lymphedema, and venous insufficiency versus other pathologies causing swelling. Additional referrals are then made to subspecialties as indicated: Lipid and Metabolism for lipedema and Vascular Specialist for venous insufficiency. Multidisciplinary team meetings help with planning, assessment, and management of lymphedema.

When diagnosed and managed at an early stage, lymphedema can be properly treated by a Certified Lymphedema Therapist (CLT) using manual therapy, compression garments, self-care, and exercise to prevent progression and ameliorate the swelling [15]. The ultimate goal in the management of lymphedema is to restore function and quality of life for the patient. When treatment is left to later stages, tissue may become fat-dominant, refractory to conservative management, and leave the patient at risk for recurrent skin infections and impaired quality of life and function.

When limb volume reduction plateaus with complete decongestive therapy, the patient is measured for a custom flat knit garment or uses a Velcro compression wrap as indicated. Simultaneously, the patient may have weight loss counseling with the endocrinology and metabolism division. If BMI is <35 and the patient is deemed a good surgical candidate after conservative management is maximized, plastic surgery may be consulted regarding debulking, lymphatic transfer surgery, and reconstruction. Decision-making about the plan of care based on the lymphedema stage is shown in Table 10.6.

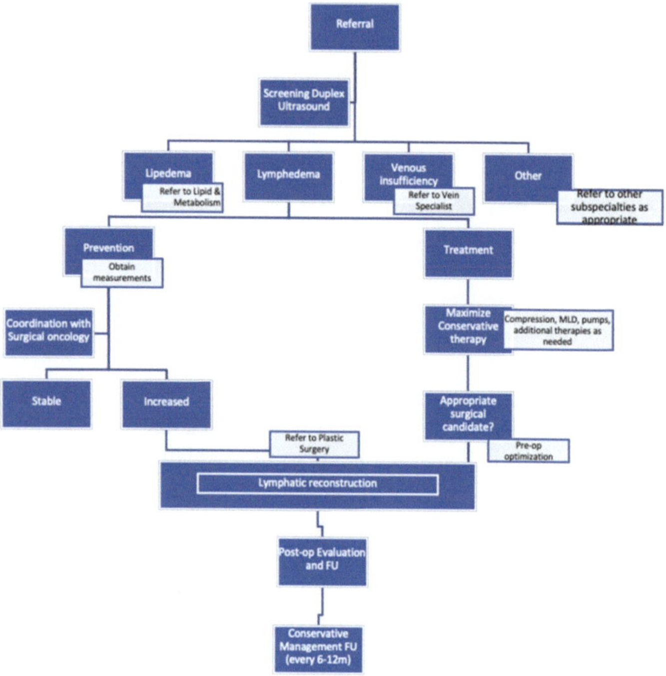

Fig. 10.5 MGH lymphatic diseases program-LERN workflow

Table 10.6 MGH protocol for managing patients with lymphedema

Stage	0	1	2	3
Diagnosis	Medical evaluation and pitting test for edema assessment			
	Lymphoscintigraphy, ICG lymphography, MRI as indicated			
Treatment	Patient education and CLT consultation			
	Stage 0: Consider compression garments especially in those at high risk; patient education, exercise, and skin care	Stage 1–3: *Phase I*: complete decongestive therapy (manuallymph drainage, multiple layer bandaging, skin care, and exercise) 3–5 days per week as indicated *Phase II:* compression garments for night and day, skin care, and exercise, consider compression pumps as adjunct to a comprehensive treatment program; Re-evaluation and updated garments every 6–12 months		
Surgery*[a]		LVA	LVA	
			VLNT	
			SAPL	SAPL
				Buried Flap

Abbreviations: *ICG* indocyanine green lymphography, *CLT* Certified Lymphedema Therapist, *LVA* lymphaticovenous anastamosis, *VLNT* vascularized lymph node transfer, *SAPL* suction-assisted protein lipectomy

[a]Consider lymphatic surgery for patients who have adhered to a course of comprehensive conservative management

Complete Decongestive Therapy (CDT) combines manual lymphatic drainage (MLD) and multi-layered bandaging to mobilize lymph fluid, in addition to skin hygiene, education, and exercise. All patients with clinical lymphedema should be offered this treatment. Phase 1 (Reduction) is intensive; visits with the CLT should occur several times per week without a gap in compression (24 h a day, 7 days a week) until limb volume reduction has plateaued; in Phase 2 (Maintenance) [33] the patient is fit for day and nighttime compression garments, and exercise progressions are taught alongside ongoing self-management education in order to maintain the benefits obtained in Phase 1. Early CDT combined with therapeutic exercise can reduce the progression of lower extremity lymphedema, improve patients' quality of life, and reduce cancer-related fatigue [93–95]. Components of conservative (non-operative) management of lymphedema are summarized in Table 10.7 [112].

Compression garments need to be replaced every 6 months and this should be part of the lymphedema management plan for long term effectiveness and safety.

Table 10.7 Components of conservative management of lymphedema

Management	Recommendations	Evidence
Skin hygiene [96]	Daily hygiene: washing with mild soap Daily application of perfume-free emollients (those containing lactic acid, urea, glycerin, ceramides, dimethicone, olive fruit oil, or salicylic acid may assist in hyperkeratotic skin desquamation) Dermatologic preparations as indicated (topical steroids, antifungals, and/or antimicrobials) Good nail hygiene	Skin disorders are a common sequela in lymphedema [96] Skin care is an important defense against infection [96]

(continued)

Table 10.7 (continued)

Management	Recommendations	Evidence
Compression: 1. Garments	Compression garments are the most important component of lymphedema management [82] Used for early stage lymphedema and during the maintenance phase of treatment for all stages Should be replaced every 6 months Garment care instructions should be followed closely to maximize effectiveness	In patients with CVD, Clinical Class 2 (USA CCL II) (30–40 mm Hg) compression stockings reduce the risk of leg ulcers, eczema, indurations, and lipodermatosclerosis compared with Clinical Class 1 or no compression [82, 97] and improve swelling severity, walking and QOL [82]. 40–60 mm Hg pressure provides the best efficacy in lower limb lymphedema [98] Appropriately fitting compression garments are the most important and impactful part of the maintenance phase of CDT, but most studies combine compression and CDT without sufficient control groups—it is difficult to draw conclusions regarding the efficacy of compression alone [82, 99] Leg compression may be considered for patients with stable CHF without decompensated heart function [100]
Compression: 2. Multiple Layer Bandaging	Used during the intensive, reduction phase of treatment Consists of clean layer against the skin, padding layer to shape and protect the limb, and compressive layer, ± toe wraps as indicated Bandages should be maintained 24 h a day throughout the reduction phase	Multilayer bandaging, followed by compression hosiery, achieves greater and more sustained limb volume reduction than hosiery alone [99].

(continued)

Table 10.7 (continued)

Management	Recommendations	Evidence
Manual Lymphatic Drainage	Used during early and later stage lymphedema Manual sequence to clear lymphatic fluid to healthy lymphatics	Manual lymphatic drainage affects the limbs and whole-body fluid composition [101] A single manual lymphatic drainage session can result in changes in both tissue dielectric constant measurements and limb girth [88, 102] Manual lymphatic drainage is usually combined with CDT in studies, making it difficult to quantify the effects of MLD alone; RCTs are needed [103]
Exercise	Physical Activity Guidelines for Americans: 150–300 min/week moderate or 75–150 min/week vigorous aerobic exercise; moderate-intensity muscles-strengthening activities at least 2 days/week, 8–15 reps for each major muscle group [104] Moderate intensity (40%–59% heart rate reserve or VO2R); vigorous intensity (60%–89% heart rate reserve or VO2R) [104]	Improves quality of life, body image/self-esteem, emotional well-being, sexuality, sleep, and social functioning; decreases: anxiety and fatigue [104, 105] Safe (when slow, gradually progressive, and supervised) and improves cardiorespiratory fitness and strength during and after cancer treatment [104, 106, 107] May decrease lower extremity lymphedema volume [107, 108] Decreases risk of cancer recurrence and treatment-related adverse effects [109]

(continued)

Table 10.7 (continued)

Management	Recommendations	Evidence
Weight management [12, 74, 110]	Losing weight (if overweight) when BMI is <50 may help improve lymphatic function, but a higher BMI may cause irreversible lymphatic damage [26, 110] Healthy weight goals should be part of a comprehensive strategy for reducing risk of chronic diseases and disease progression	BMI >30 increases risk of lymphedema, BMI of 50–60 incurs very high risk [110, 111]

Safety Considerations During Fluid Mobilization in Lymphedema Treatment and Follow-Up

Systemic pathology must first be managed. Every patient planning compression therapy should be screened for conditions that increase the risk of complications [100]. Fluid shifts must be considered when dealing with patients with congestive heart failure or COPD. The CLT needs to know how much fluid can safely be returned to the heart [113]. Tolerance for CDT should be monitored with: hemodynamic assessment at rest and with activity, pulmonary auscultation, repeat measurement of lower extremity volume, dyspnea rating (Borg scale), functional tests (6 Minute Walk Test, Timed Up & Go, Gait speed, vital signs -BP, HR, O2sat-) and monitoring for paroxysmal nocturnal dyspnea. The vascular specialist should rule out arterial disease (cold skin, decreased pedal pulses, delayed capillary refill) or abnormal ABI. In severe peripheral artery occlusive disease, sustained non-elastic compression is contraindicated if the systolic ankle pressure is <60 mmHg or the toe pressure is <30 mmHg [82, 100].

Pneumatic Compression Devices, as an adjunct to traditional conservative management, may help improve leg circumference, bioimpedance measurements, and pain in patients with lymphedema and lipedema [114]. However, this is an adjunct to a comprehensive treatment program and is not to be used as a stand-alone intervention. As with multilayered bandaging for CDT, precautions for mobilizing large amounts of stagnant lower extremity fluid to return it to central circulation should first be understood for those with cardiac, renal, or hepatic issues.

Lymphatic Surgeries are emerging as either preventative treatments at the time of definitive lymph node removal or for those whose lymphedema is refractory to conservative measures. Surgeries are either *physiologic* (lymphovenous bypass and vascularized lymph node transplant to improve lymphatic drainage) or *excisional* ("debulking" by suction-assisted lipectomy or direct excisional procedures to reduce the lymphedema-related load). They are not curative but can improve symptoms, lymphatic function, and QOL for some patients with primary and secondary lower extremity lymphedema alongside compression therapy and exercise [2, 26, 115]. Referral to lymphatic surgery should be considered in all patients in which node dissection is planned so that they can be evaluated for lymphatic microsurgical preventing healing approach (LYMPHA), in which disrupted lymphatics are immediately placed within adjacent veins for lymphovenous bypass to prevent the development of lymphedema in that high-risk group. It should be noted that lymphatic surgery is typically not offered for lymphedema when BMI > 35 kg/m^2; emphasis should be placed on weight management with subsequent lymphatic surgery referral. Several evidence-based algorithms are available in the literature to guide decision-making, such as the *Algorithm of lymphedema clinical stage and corresponding operative management of lower extremity lymphedema* [116] within Ramachandran et al. [116] and the *Patients with chronic lymphedema: flow and work-up through the lymphatic center* [117] described in the Granoff et al. study: *A Single Institution Multidisciplinary Approach to Power-Assisted Liposuction for the Management of Lymphedema* [117].

For patients who have already entered a proliferative phase of lymphedema, in which their extremities have become fat dominant rather than fluid dominant in terms of clinical and radiologic appearance, debulking with large-volume liposuction is done first, followed by compression therapy. It should be noted that this type of liposuction is not cosmetic and is completed with specialized tools to help prevent damage to the lymphatic system. After 1 year, consideration for physiologic reconstruction is then given. There is some disagreement about the proper sequence or combination of debulking and physiologic surgical intervention, and future clinical series will help better determine the optimal approach, which is evolving.

Key Point Synopsis

Lymphedema can be detected on clinical exam in patients with measurable swelling and skin changes; however it can be more difficult to diagnose in patients who report limb heaviness or fullness but without clinically detectable limb volume change or other symptoms. Therefore, the diagnosis of lymphedema depends on the integration of patient-reported symptoms, clinical examination, and objective measurements. Medical testing to clarify potential underlying etiologies is important, as not all lower extremity swelling is lymphedema, and lymphedema can coexist with other sources of swelling. Prospective screening of symptoms and objective measurements preoperatively in the context of cancer treatments and at regular intervals postoperatively should be available to all patients at risk of lymphedema. Early stage lymphedema is the most responsive to conservative management compared to later stages, and early detection and treatment should be the goal. Later-stage lymphedema may require additional surgical interventions to physiologically improve the affected extremity by offering improved lymphatic outflow or to lower the burden of disease with direct debulking with liposuction. Lymphedema is a lifelong disease that is not curable. Therefore, early and ongoing consultations with a lymphedema specialist at regular intervals within the context of a multidisciplinary screening and treatment program are imperative for early diagnosis, management, and prevention of lymphedema progression in order to maximize patient QOL and optimize short- and long-term outcomes.

Summary

Lymphedema is a chronic, progressive disease affecting millions of people worldwide, but it is often overlooked. Protein-rich fluid accumulates in the interstitial space due to either primary congenital disease or secondary damage to the lymphatic system, often associated with surgery or cancer treatments. Comparing and contrasting the presentation of lymphedema-related lower extremity swelling with other etiologies and clinical presentations will illuminate accurate differential diagnosis. Timely diagnosis of lymphedema and proper management are key to avoiding loss of function, disfigurement, pain, and decreased quality of life.

References

1. Gasparis AP, Kim PS, Dean SM, Khilnani NM, Labropoulos N. Diagnostic approach to lower limb edema. Phlebology. 2020;35(9):650–5.
2. Schaverien M, Coroneos C. Surgical treatment of lymphedema. Plast Reconstr Surg. 2019;144(3):738–58.
3. Russo S, Walker JL, Carlson JW, Carter J. Standardization of lower extremity quantitative lymphedema measurements and associated patient-reported outcomes in gynecologic cancers. Gynecol Oncol. 2021;160(2):625–32. Published online 2020.
4. Lymphatic Education and Research Network. The incidence and prevalence of lymphedema. Accessed 18 Nov 2023. https://lymphaticnetwork.org/living-with-lymphedema/the-incidence-of-lymphedema#:~:text=Up%20to%20250%20million%20people,5%2C%20and%20ALS6%20combined.
5. Bianchi LMG, Irmici G, Cè M, et al. Diagnosis and treatment of post-prostatectomy lymphedema: what's new? Curr Oncol. 2023;30(5):4512–26.
6. Moffatt CJ, Aubeeluck A, Franks PJ, et al. Psychological factors in chronic edema: a case-control study. Lymphat Res Biol. 2017;15:252–61.
7. Mathevet P, Lécuru F, Uzan C, Boutitie F, Magaud L, Guyon F, Querleu D, Fourchotte V, Baron M, Bats A-S, Senticol 2 Group. Sentinel lymph node biopsy for early cervical cancer: results of a randomized prospective, multicenter study (SENTICOL 2) comparing adding pelvic lymph node dissection vs. sentinel node biopsy only. Gynecol Oncol. 2017;145(1):2–3.

8. Carlsson S, Bottai M, Lantz A, Bjartell A, Hugosson J, Steineck G, Stranne J, Wiklund P, Haglind E, Akre O. Lymph swelling after radical prostatectomy and pelvic lymph node dissection. BJU Int. 2022;129:695–8.
9. Földi M, Földi E, Strößenreuther R, Kubik S. Földi's textbook of lymphology: for physicians and lymphedema therapists. 3rd ed. San Francisco: Urban & Fischer; 2012.
10. Carlson J, Kauderer J, Hutson A. GOG 244 – the lymphedema and gynecologic cancer (LEG) study: incidence and risk factors in newly diagnosed patients. Gynecol Oncol. 2020;156:467–74.
11. Banner L, Cohen A, Patel V, Nikbakht N. A practical approach to the diagnosis of lymphedema: a narrative review. Dermatol Pract Concept. 2023;13(3):e2023132.
12. Greene A, Goss J. Diagnosis and staging of lymphedema. Semin Plast Surg. 2018;32(1):12–6.
13. Rockson SG. Lymphedema. Am J Med. 2001;110:288–95.
14. Tada H, Teramukai S, Fukushima M, Sasaki H. Risk factors for lower limb lymphedema after lymph node dissection in patients with ovarian and uterine carcinoma. BMC Cancer. 2009;9:47.
15. Clinckaert A, Callens K, Cooreman A, et al. The prevalence of lower limb and genital lymphedema after prostate cancer treatment: a systematic review. Cancers (Basel). 2022;14:5667.
16. McDonagh T, Metra M, Adamo M, et al. 2021 ESC Guidelines for the diagnosis and treatment of acute and chronic heart failure. Task Force for the diagnosis and treatment of acute and chronic heart failure of the European Society of Cardiology (ESC) with the special contribution of the Heart Failure Association (HFA) of the ESC. Published online 27 Jan 2022.
17. Del Buono MG, Arena R, Borlaug BA, Carbone S, Canada JM, Kirkman DL, Garten R, Rodriguez-Miguelez P, Guazzi M, Lavie CJ, Abbate A. Exercise intolerance in patients with heart failure: JACC state-of-the-art review. J Am Coll Cardiol. 2019;73(17):2209–25.
18. Pieske B, Tschöpe C, de Boer RA, et al. How to diagnose heart failure with preserved ejection fraction: the HFA–PEFF diagnostic algorithm: a consensus recommendation from the Heart Failure Association (HFA) of the European Society of Cardiology (ESC). Eur Heart J. 2019;40(40):3297–317.
19. Odak M, Kayani W. MUGA scan. In: StatPearls [Internet]. Treasure Island (FL): StatPearls Publishing; 2023. Published online 25 July 2023.
20. Baumgarten M, Gehr TWB, Kothari NR, Carl D. Diseases of the kidney. In: Paulman PM, Taylor RB, Paulman AA, Nasir LS, editors. Family medicine. Cham: Springer; 2022.
21. Narva A, Bilous R. Laboratory assessment of diabetic kidney disease. Diabetes Spectr. 2015;28(3):162–6.

22. Koo H, Hwang S, Kim T, et al. The ratio of urinary sodium and potassium and chronic kidney disease progression: results from the Korean Cohort Study for Outcomes in Patients with Chronic Kidney Disease. Medicine. 2018;97(44):12820.
23. Vaidya, Satyanarayana R, Aeddula NR. Chronic kidney disease. In: NCBI Bookshelf. A Service of the National Library of Medicine, National Institutes of Health. StatPearls [Internet]. StatPearls Publishing; 2022.
24. Heidelbaugh J, Bruderly M. Cirrhosis and chronic liver failure: part I. Diagnosis and evaluation. Am Fam Physician. 2006;74(5):756–62.
25. Eberhardt RT, Raffetto JD. Chronic venous insufficiency. Circulation. 2014;130(4):333–46.
26. Sudduth C, Greene A. Primary lymphedema: update on genetic basis and management. Adv Wound Care. 2022;11(7):374–81.
27. Smeltzer D, Stickler G, Schirger A. Primary lymphedema in children and adolescents: a follow-up study and review. Pediatrics. 1985;76(2):206–18.
28. Lee B, Andrade M, Bergan J, et al. Diagnosis and treatment of primary lymphedema. Consensus Document of the International Union of Phlebology (IUP). Int Union Phlebol. 2009;29(5):454–70.
29. Lee BB, Andrade M, Bergen J, et al. Diagnosis and treatment of primary lymphedema. Consensus Document of the International Union of Phlebology (IUP)-2009. Int Angiol. 2010;29(4):454–70.
30. Vignes S. Lymphedema: from diagnosis to treatment. Rev Med Interne. 2017;38(2):97–105.
31. Bianchi L, Irmici G, Ce M. Diagnosis and treatment of post-prostatectomy lymphedema: what's new? Curr Oncol. 2023;30(5):4512–26.
32. Centers for Disease Control and Prevention. Parasites – lymphatic filariasis. https://www.cdc.gov/parasites/lymphaticfilariasis/index.html.
33. Chang D, Masia J, Garza R, Skoracki R, Neligan P. Lymphedema: surgical and medical therapy. Plast Reconstr Surg. 2016;138:209S–18S.
34. Ancukiewicz M, Miller C, Skolny M, et al. Comparison of relative versus absolute arm size change as criteria for quantifying breast cancer-related lymphedema: the flaws in current studies and need for universal methodology. Erratum in: Breast Cancer Res Treat. 2012;136(2):623.
35. Brunelle C, Roberts S, Horick N, et al. Integrating symptoms into the diagnostic criteria for breast cancer-related lymphedema: applying results from a prospective surveillance program. Phys Ther. 2020;100(12):2186–97.
36. Brunelle C, Roberts SA, Horick NK, et al. Integrating symptoms into the diagnostic criteria for breast cancer-related lymphedema: applying results from a prospective surveillance program. Phys Ther. 2000;100(12):2186–97.

37. Sun F, Skolny M, Swaroop M, et al. The need for preoperative baseline arm measurement to accurately quantify breast cancer-related lymphedema. Breast Cancer Res Treat. 2016;157:229–40.
38. Cavezzi A, Urso S, Paccasassi S, Mosti G, Campana F, Colucci R. Bioimpedance spectroscopy and volumetry in the immediate/short-term monitoring of intensive complex decongestive treatment of lymphedema. Phlebology. 2020;35(9):715–23.
39. Jeffers EJ, Wagner JL, Korentager SS, et al. Breast cancer-related lymphedema (BCRL) and bioimpedance spectroscopy: long-term follow-up, surveillance recommendations, and multidisciplinary risk factors. Ann Surg Oncol. 2023;30:6258–65.
40. Forner-Cordero I. Update in the management of lipedema. Int Angiol. 2021;40(4):345–57.
41. Lohrmann C, Foeldi E, Langer M. MR imaging of the lymphatic system in patients with lipedema and lipo-lymphedema. Microvasc Res. 2009;77(3):335–9. ISSN 0026-2862.
42. Kalawat T, Reddy P, Suneetha B. Role of lymphoscintigraphy in diagnosis and management of patients with leg swelling of unclear etiology. Indian J Nucl Med. 2012;27(4):226–30.
43. Palanisamy D, Omkumar A. A study on the effectiveness of wells criteria for diagnosing deep vein thrombosis: a prospective observational study. Int Surg J. 2021;8(2):569–74.
44. Modi S, Dealer R, Gozel K. Wells criteria for DVT is a reliable clinical tool to assess the risk of deep venous thrombosis in trauma patients. World J Emerg Surg. 2016;11(24):1–6.
45. Togale M, Gupta P. Study to determine Wells criteria as a reliable clinical tool in diagnosis of deep vein thrombosis: a one year cross-sectional single centric hospital based study. Int Surg J. 2021;8(12):3634–8.
46. Warwick D, Nadia R. The "critical thrombosis period" in major orthopedic surgery: when to start and when to stop prophylaxis. Clin Appl Thromb Hemost. 2010;16(4):394–405.
47. Pua YH. The time course of knee swelling post total knee arthroplasty and its associations with quadriceps strength and gait speed. J Arthroplast. 2015;30(7):1215–9.
48. Szöts K, Pedersen PU, Hørdam B, Thomsen T, Konradsen H. Physical health problems experienced in the early postoperative recovery period following total knee replacement. Int J Orthop Trauma Nurs. 2015;19(1):36–44.
49. Kwok F, Zaya S, Moorchilot R, Shah A. Case of unilateral leg swelling: a DVT mimic. BMJ Case Rep. 2018;2018:bcr2017221651. Published online 18 May 2018.
50. Heart.org. Medication used to treat heart failure. https://www.heart.org/en/health-topics/heart-failure/treatment-options-for-heart-failure/medications-used-to-treat-heart-failure.

51. Makani H, Bangalore S, Romero J, et al. Peripheral edema associated with calcium channel blockers: incidence and withdrawal rate—a meta-analysis of randomized trials. J Hypertens. 2011;29(7):1270–80.
52. Skovbjerg B, Helgestad O, Oxlund C, Christensen B, Henriksen J. Management of amlodipine-induced ankle oedema. Ugeskr Laeger Danish. 2023;185(16):V07220460.
53. Largeau B, Cracowski JL, Lengellé C, Sautenet B, Jonville-Béra AP. Drug-induced peripheral oedema: an aetiology-based review. Br J Clin Pharmacol. 2021;87(8):3043–55.
54. Daniell K, Bardia A, Sun F, et al. Incidence of peripheral edema in patients receiving PI3K/mTOR/CDK4/6 inhibitors for metastatic breast cancer. Breast Cancer Res Treat. 2019;175(3):649–58.
55. Salani R, Preston M, Hade E, Johns J, Fowler J, Paskett E. Swelling among women who need education about leg lymphedema: a descriptive study of lymphedema in women undergoing surgery for endometrial cancer. Int J Gynecol Cancer. 2014;24:1507–12.
56. Raskin Y, Jorissen C, Joniau S, Everaerts W. MP54-17 The prevalence, risk factors and impact on quality of life of lymphedema after robot-assisted radical prostatectomy with extended pelvic lymph node dissection. J Urol. 2019;201(4). https://doi.org/10.1097/01.JU.0000556678.70718.d6.
57. Woon PC, Kim I, Kim JH, Hwang JH. Association of clinical manifestations of secondary lymphedema and lymph node dissection sites in the lower extremities of patients with melanoma. Acta Oncol (Madr). 2023;62(8):880–8.
58. Hyngstrom JR, Chiang YJ, Cromwell KD, et al. Prospective assessment of lymphedema incidence and lymphedema-associated symptoms following lymph node surgery for melanoma. Melanoma Res. 2013;23(4):290–7.
59. Hu H, Fu M, Huang X, Huang J, Gao J. Risk factors for lower extremity lymphedema after cervical cancer treatment: a systematic review and meta-analysis. Transl Cancer Res. 2022;11(6):1713–21.
60. Bae H, Lim M, Lee J, Lee Y, Nam B, Seo S. Postoperative lower extremity edema in patients with primary endometrial cancer. Ann Surg Oncol. 2016;23(1):186–95. Published online 2016.
61. Carter J, Huang H, Armer J, et al. The LymphEdema and Gynecologic cancer (LEG) study: the association between the gynecologic cancer lymphedema questionnaire (GCLQ) and lymphedema of the lower extremity (LLE). Gynecol Oncol. 2019;155(3):452–60.
62. Yost K, Cheville A, Weaver A, Hilli M, Dowdy S. Development and validation of a self-report lower-extremity lymphedema screening questionnaire in women. Phys Ther. 2013;93(5):694–703.
63. Ridner S, Doersam J, Stolldorf D, Dietrich M. Development and validation of the lymphedema symptom intensity and distress survey-lower limb. Lymphat Res Bio. 2018;16(6):538–46.

64. Dellino G, Kaminsky T, Tomlin G. Review of health-related quality of life assessments for patients with lymphedema. Am J Occup Ther. 2018;72(4):1.
65. Xu C, Christensen JM, Haykal T, Asaad M, Sidey-Gibbons C, Schaverien M. Measurement properties of the lymphedema life impact scale. Lymphat Res Biol. 2022;20(4):425–34.
66. Coriddi M, Kim L, McGrath L, et al. Accuracy, sensitivity, and specificity of the LLIS and ULL27 in detecting breast cancer-related lymphedema. Ann Surg Oncol. 2022;29:438–45.
67. Wedin M, Fredrikson M, Ahlner E, et al. Validation of the Lymphoedema Quality of Life Questionnaire (LYMQOL) in Swedish cancer patients. Acta Oncol. 2020;59(3):365–71.
68. Addiss D, Armer J, Billingham R. In: Moffatt C, Doherty D, Morgan P, editors. Lymphedema framework: best practice for the management of lymphedema – international consensus. London: Medical Education Partnership, Ltd; 2006.
69. Seidel H, Ball J, Dains J. Mosby's guide to physical examination. 7th ed. St. Louis: Elsevier; 2011.
70. O'Sullivan SB, Schmitz TJ, Fulk GD. Physical rehabilitation: assessment and treatment. Philadelphia: F.A. Davis Co.; 2014.
71. Sanderson J, Tuttle N, Box R, Reul-Hirche H, Laakso E. The pitting test: an investigation of an unstandardized assessment of lymphedema. Lymphology. 2015;48:175–83.
72. Stemmer R. Stemmer's sign: possibilities and limits of clinical diagnosis of lymphedema. Wien Med Wochenschr. 1999;149:85–6.
73. Stemmer R. A clinical symptom for the early and differential diagnosis of lymphedema. Vasa. 1976;5:261–2.
74. Goss J, Greene A. Sensitivity and specificity of the Stemmer sign for lymphedema: a clinical lymphoscintigraphic study. Plast Reconstr Surg Glob Open. 2019;7(6):2295.
75. Osman AA, Ju W, Sun D, Qi B. Deep venous thrombosis: a literature review. Int J Clin Exp Med. 2018;11(3):1551–61.
76. Taylor R, Jayasinghe U, Koelmeyer L, Ung O, Boyages J. Reliability and validity of arm volume measurements for assessment of lymphedema. Phys Ther. 2006;86(2):205–14.
77. Ancukiewicz M, Russell T, Otoole J, et al. Standardized method for quantification of developing lymphedema in patients treated for breast cancer. Int J Radiat Oncol Biol Phys. 2011;79(5):1436–43.
78. Stanton A, Northfield J, Holroyd B. Validation of an optoelectronic limb volumeter (Perometer). Lymphology. 1997;30:77–97.
79. Lee M, Boland R, Czerniec S, Kilbreath S. Reliability and concurrent validity of the perometer for measuring hand volume in women with and without lymphedema. Lymphat Res Biol. 2011;9:13–8.
80. Schonholz S. Preoperative assessment enables the early detection and successful treatment of lymphedema. Cancer. 2009;115:909.

81. Hidding J, Viehoff P, Beurskens C, van Laarhoven H, Nihjhuis-van der Sanden M, van der Wees P. Measurement properties of instruments for measuring of lymphedema: systematic review. Phys Ther. 2016;96:1965–81.
82. Rabe E, Partsch H, Hafner J, et al. Indications for medical compression stockings in venous and lymphatic disorders: an evidence-based consensus statement. Phlebology. 2018;33(3):163–84.
83. Ward L, Winall A, Isenring E, et al. Assessment of bilateral limb lymphedema by bioelectrical impedance spectroscopy. Int J Gynecol Cancer. 2011;21(2):409–18.
84. Barrio A, Eaton A, Frazier T. A prospective validation study of bioimpedance with volume displacement in early-stage breast cancer patients at risk for lymphedema. Ann Surg Oncol. 2015;22(3):370–5.
85. Lahtinen T, Seppälä J, Viren T, Johansson K. Experimental and analytical comparisons of tissue dielectric constant (TDC) and bioimpedance spectroscopy (BIS) in assessment of early arm lymphedema in breast cancer patients after axillary surgery and radiotherapy. Lymphat Res Biol. 2015;13(3):176–85.
86. Bundred N, Stockton C, Keeley V, et al. Investigators of BEA/PLACE studies, Comparison of multi-frequency bioimpedance with perometry for the early detection and intervention of lymphoedema after axillary node clearance for breast cancer. Breast Cancer Res Treat. 2015;151(1):121–9.
87. Qin ES, Bowen MJ, Chen WF. Diagnostic accuracy of bioimpedance spectroscopy in patients with lymphedema: a retrospective cohort analysis. J Plast Reconstr Aesthet Surg. 2018;71(7):1041–50.
88. Mayrovitz HN. Tissue dielectric constant of the lower leg as an index of skin water: temporal variations. Cureus. 2022;14(7):e26506.
89. Herbst KL, Kahn LA, Iker E, et al. Standard of care for lipedema in the United States. Phlebology. 2021;36(10):779–96.
90. Herbst K. Rare adipose disorders (RADs) masquerading as obesity. Acta Pharmacol Sin. 2012;33(2):155–72.
91. Bertsch T, Erbacher G, Elwell R. Lipoedema: a paradigm shift and consensus. J Wound Care. 2020;29(Sup11b):1–51.
92. Coppel T, Cunneen J, Fetzer S, Gordon K, Hardy D, Jones K, et al. Best practice guidelines: the management of lipoedema. Wounds UK. Published online 2017. Accessed 20 July 2024. https://wounds-uk.com/wp-content/uploads/sites/2/2023/02/450f55130cff87901188206fd115ccf3.pdf.
93. Noh S, Hwang J, Yoon T, Chang H, Chu I, Kim J. Limb differences in the therapeutic effects of complex decongestive therapy on edema, quality of life, and satisfaction in lymphedema patients. Ann Rehabil Med. 2015;39(3):347–59.

94. Cobbe S, Nugent K, Real S. Pilot study: the effectiveness of complex decongestive therapy for lymphedema in palliative care patients with advanced cancer. J Palliat Med. 2018;21(4):473–8.
95. Wu X, Liu Y, Zhu D, Wang F, Ji J, Yan H. Early prevention of complex decongestive therapy and rehabilitation exercise for prevention of lower extremity lymphedema after operation of gynecologic cancer. Asian J Surg. 2021;44(1):111–5.
96. Fife CE, Farrow W, Hebert AA, et al. Skin and wound care in lymphedema patients: a taxonomy, primer, and literature review. Adv Skin Wound Care. 2017;30(7):305–18.
97. Dahm K, Myrhaug H, Strømme H. Effects of preventive use of compression stockings for elderly with chronic venous insufficiency and swollen legs: a systematic review and meta-analysis. BMC Geriatr. 2019;7(19):76.
98. Mosti G, Cavezzi A. Compression therapy in lymphedema: between past and recent scientific data. Phlebology. 2019;34(8):515–22.
99. Badger C, Peacock J, Mortimer P. A randomized, controlled, parallel-group clinical trial comparing multilayer bandaging followed by hosiery versus hosiery alone in the treatment of patients with lymphedema of the limb. Cancer. 2000;88(12):2832–7.
100. Rabe E, Partsch H, Morrison N, et al. Risks and contraindications of medical compression treatment – a critical reappraisal. An international consensus statement. Phlebology. 2020;35(7):447–60.
101. Brix B, Apich G, Roessler A, et al. Fluid shifts induced by physical therapy in lower limb lymphedema patients. J Clin Med. 2020;9:3678.
102. Mayrovitz HN, Davey S, Shapiro E. Localized tissue water changes accompanying one manual lymphatic drainage (MLD) therapy session assessed by changes in tissue dielectric constant in patients with lower extremity lymphedema. Lymphology. 2008;41:87–92.
103. Moffatt CJ, Burian E, Karlsmark T, et al. Factors predicting limb volume reduction using compression bandaging within decongestive lymphatic therapy in lymphedema: a multicountry prospective study. Lymphat Res Biol. 2021;19(5):412–22.
104. Campbell KL, Winter-Stone KM, Wiskemann J, et al. Exercise guidelines for cancer survivors: consensus statement from international multidisciplinary roundtable. Med Sci Sports Exerc. 2019;51(11):2375–90.
105. Mishra S, Scherer R, Geigle P, et al. Exercise interventions on health-related quality of life for cancer survivors. Cochrane Database Syst Rev 2012. 2013;8.
106. Schmitz KH, Campbell AM, Stuiver MM, et al. Exercise is medicine in oncology: engaging clinicians to help patients move through cancer. A A Cancer J Clin. 2019;69:468–84. https://doi.org/10.3322/caac.21579.
107. Do JH, Choi KH, Ahn JS, Jeon JY. Effects of a complex rehabilitation program on edema status, physical function, and quality of life in lower-

limb lymphedema after gynecological cancer surgery. Gynecol Oncol. 2017;147:45–455.

108. Brown J, John G, Segal S, Chu C, Schmitz K. Physical activity and lower limb lymphedema among uterine cancer survivors. Med Sci Sports Exerc. 2013;45(11):2091–7.
109. Cormie P, Zopf EM, Zhang X, Schmitz KH. The impact of exercise on cancer mortality, recurrence, and treatment-related adverse effects. Epidemiol Rev. 2017;1:71–92.
110. Sudduth C, Greene A. Current overview of obesity-induced lymphedema. Adv Wound Care (New Rochelle). 2022;11(7):392–8.
111. O'Malley E, Ahern T, Dunlevy C, Lehane C, Kirby B, O'Shea D. Obesity-related chronic lymphoedema-like swelling and physical function. QJM. 2015;108(3):183–7.
112. Executive Committee. The diagnosis and treatment of peripheral lymphedema: 2016 consensus document of the International Society of Lymphology. Lymphology. 2016;49(4):170–84.
113. Vaassen M. Manual lymph drainage in a patient with congestive heart failure: a case study. Ostomy Wound Manage. 2015;6(10):38–45.
114. Wright T, Scarfino C, O'Malley E. Effect of pneumatic compression device and stocking use on symptoms and quality of life in women with lipedema: a proof-in-principle randomized trial. Phlebology. 2023;38(1):51–61.
115. Shaitelman S, Cromwell K, Rasmussen J. Recent progress in the treatment and prevention of cancer-related lymphedema. CA Cancer J Clin. 2015;65:55–81.
116. Ramachandran S, Chew K, Tan B, Kuo Y. Current operative management and therapeutic algorithm of lymphedema in the lower extremities. Asian J Surg. 2021;44(1):46–53.
117. Granoff M, Johnson A, Shillue K, et al. A single institution multi-disciplinary approach to power-assisted liposuction for the management of lymphedema. Ann Surg. 2022;276(5):e613–21.

Part V

Protocols

Duplex Ultrasound of the Lower Limb: Deep System

11

Ryan T. Brooks and Anahita Dua

Purpose

To evaluate for the presence of venous thrombosis in the lower extremities. This study should also include assessment of the great and small saphenous veins for superficial thrombus.

R. T. Brooks (✉) · A. Dua
Division of Vascular and Endovascular Surgery, Department of Surgery, Massachusetts General Hospital/Harvard Medical School, Boston, MA, USA
e-mail: rtbrooks@mgh.harvard.edu; adua1@mgh.harvard.edu

C. Echevarria et al. (eds.), *The Massachusetts General Hospital Protocols and Procedures for Venous Disease*, https://doi.org/10.1007/978-3-032-05708-2_11

Indications

Include but are not limited to.

- Leg swelling
- Leg pain
- Shortness of breath
- Tenderness
- Palpable Cord
- Status Post Venous Ablation
- New lower extremity pain while on Anticoagulation
- Before terminating anticoagulation therapy [1]

Preparation

None needed

Equipment

General Electric E10

- L2-9 Probe
- C1-6 Probe
- IC5-9 Probe
- L8-18 Probe

Ultrasound gel
Cloth towels
Transducer cleaner

Patient History and Positioning

A patient history is obtained and should include presenting symptoms and risk factors, with physical examination performed to assess for leg pain and swelling.

The patient is placed supinely, with the leg to be examined externally rotated.

Technique

Transverse compression should be considered the primary method of determining the presence or absence of thrombus in the veins. The vein should be viewed in the transverse plane, with compressing applied every 2 cm.

Color and/or spectral Doppler are used to determine the presence and characteristics of the flow within the veins.

Procedure

1. Examination starts with a transverse view of the common femoral vein (CFV)/saphenofemoral junction in B-mode. Compression maneuvers of the CFV are performed proximal to the inguinal canal, at the SFJ, and just distal to the inguinal canal. The transducer is rotated 90° into longitudinal view and a spectral Doppler waveform of the common femoral vein is obtained to assess character of flow.
2. The transducer is rotated 90° and B-mode compression images of the femoral vein start just below the inguinal ligament and move distally, with compressions every 2 cm. The femoral vein is examined in this fashion from the proximal thigh to the adductor canal. When visualized, the proximal profunda femoris vein is to be documented with and without compression maneuvers. The transducer is then returned to the saphenofemoral junction, and the great saphenous vein is examined for compressibility. Transverse compressions of

the greater saphenous vein are done from the saphenofemoral junction to the ankle.

3. The transducer is then placed into the popliteal fossa, and the popliteal, gastrocnemius, and small saphenous veins are examined. To facilitate imaging of the calf veins, the patient may be put in slight reverse Trendelenburg's position, or the knee may be bent upward to facilitate pooling of venous blood in the calf.
4. A Doppler sample of the popliteal vein at rest is obtained.
5. The transducer is rotated 90°. Transverse compressions start as proximally as possible in the popliteal vein, moving along its length, with compressions every 2 cm.
6. The gastrocnemius veins (medial and lateral) are also examined for compressibility.
7. The small saphenous vein is examined for compression from the knee area to the ankle, if the vein is large enough.
8. The transducer is then placed in a transverse orientation at the ankle. The posterior tibial veins are examined for compressibility from the ankle to the tibial-peroneal trunk/distal popliteal vein.
9. The peroneal veins are identified in a similar manner with transverse compressions along their lengths. If necessary to obtain adequate images, the peroneal veins may be examined from a lateral or posterolateral approach.
10. Due to the very low incidence of isolated anterior tibial vein thrombosis, examination of those veins may be limited to cases in which there has been trauma localized to the anterior lower leg.
11. Calf muscle branches, including gastrocnemius and soleal veins, are assessed for incompressibility.
12. At the end of the procedure, if the patient complains of a specific area of discomfort that has not been examined, that area should then be examined for the presence of thrombus.
13. All incidental findings should be imaged and mentioned in the technologist's report.

NOTE: If a unilateral study has been ordered, examination of the contralateral common femoral vein should be done to assess for compression and phasicity, to compare right and left common femoral Doppler signals, as specified by IAC standards.

Saved Images for a Normal Study

Doppler

1. Common femoral vein at the saphenofemoral junction demonstrating spontaneity, and phasicity bilaterally.
2. Popliteal vein demonstrating spontaneity.

Grayscale Images (May Be Done with Split-Screen View)

1. Transverse view of the common femoral vein at the saphenofemoral junction, with and without compression.
2. Transverse view of the femoral vein at proximal, mid, and distal thigh levels, with and without compression.
3. Transverse view of the popliteal vein, with and without compression.
4. Transverse view of the deep calf veins (posterior tibial, gastrocnemius, and peroneal), with and without compression.

Saved Images for a Positive Study

Where thrombus is clearly visualized within a vein, compressions may be omitted to minimize the risk of embolization of thrombus. If thrombus is difficult to document due to echo lucent nature of the thrombus, gentle compression may be done to show abnormal response; however, utmost care should be exercised to apply only enough pressure to cause vein walls to come into gentle contact with the intraluminal thrombus. Pulsed-wave Doppler waveforms are to be obtained at the site of the thrombus to document absence of flow or diminished flow. Color Doppler may also be used to show absence of color filling in the affected area. Distal augmentation is to be omitted in the presence of visualized thrombus to minimize the risk of embolization.

Grayscale and Spectral Doppler Images for a Positive Study

1. Transverse view of the thrombosed vein, with and without compression.
2. Anatomical locations of all thrombosed vessels with physical landmarks when possible.
3. When possible, a longitudinal measurement of the length of the thrombosed vessel.
4. Pulsed-wave Doppler waveforms to be obtained at the site of the thrombus to document absence of flow or diminished flow around thrombus.
5. When superficial thrombus is identified, the distance from the most proximal portion of the thrombus to the SFJ or SPJ is to be documented.

Interpretation for a Normal Study

- Imaging—Veins should fully compress, with no evidence of echogenic material.
- Doppler—Blood flow should demonstrate normal lower-extremity venous flow characteristics as described below [1].

  SPONTANEITY

  Flow should be present in the larger, more proximal veins at rest but may not be present in more distal veins of the leg; manual compression may be needed to demonstrate its presence.

  PHASICITY

  Absence of phasicity or asymmetrical phasicity when comparing waveforms within the bilateral common femoral veins may represent a more proximal obstruction—extrinsic or intrinsic.

PULSATILITY

Normal lower-extremity venous signals are non-pulsatile. The presence of pulsatile flow may indicate venous hypertension.

AUGMENTATION

Augmentation is not required during assessment of the deep veins and should only be done to demonstrate flow in a vessel that cannot be compressed due to patient discomfort or body habitus. Manual compression of the extremity distal to the site being examined with Doppler should cause an increase in blood flow. Failure to do so, or a weak response, may represent an obstruction between the site being examined and the site of manual compression.

Interpretation for a Positive Study

- IMAGING

  The vein is commonly dilated in an acute obstruction, noncompressible, and contains lightly echogenic material, although echogenicity has been shown to be an unreliable indicator of the age of venous thrombosis. Whenever possible, the tip of the thrombus should be examined in a longitudinal plane and assessed for mobility and attachment to the vein wall.

  Acute thrombus often appears "homogenous/hypoechoic" and may be occlusive, with the partly occlusive tip in the middle of the lumen.

  With a chronic obstruction, the vein may be small and retracted, and/or contain brightly echogenic material that is often partly occlusive. Grayscale examination in the longitudinal plane demonstrates firm, well-attached material without a "bullet-shaped" tip.

  Any critical findings are to be immediately relayed to the ordering provider, who will then instruct the patient on treatment procedures. If an exam is ordered by an outside provider,

all critical findings will be relayed to them and the study will be read out within 24 h.
The technologist will document that critical findings were conveyed to the reading provider or referring provider under the "Findings" section of the report.

- SPECTRAL DOPPLER/COLOR FLOW
  Blood flow will be absent in a totally occluded vein, with some flow present in a partially obstructed vein. Loss of spontaneous phasic flow may represent a more proximal obstruction—via extrinsic compression or intrinsic obtruction of the venous system.
- INCIDENTAL FINDINGS
  All incidental findings should be included in the final interpretation.

Summary

This chapter details the technical aspects of evaluation of the deep and superficial venous system. Here we detail the patient selection, equipment, and technical aspects of the exam. We also describe in detail the appropriate actions for a positive study. Where thrombus is clearly visualized within a vein, compression may be omitted to minimize the risk of embolization of thrombus. If thrombus is difficult to document due to the echolucent nature of the thrombus, gentle compression may be done to show abnormal response; however, utmost care should be exercised to apply only enough pressure to cause vein walls to come into gentle contact with the intraluminal thrombus. Pulsed Wave Doppler waveforms are to be obtained at the site of the thrombus to document absence of flow or diminished flow. Color Doppler may also be used to show absence of color filling in the affected area. Distal augmentation is to be omitted in the presence of visualized thrombus to minimize the risk of embolization.

References

1. Society for Vascular Ultrasound. SVU Vascular Technology Professional Performance Guidelines. Lower Extremity Venous Duplex Evaluation. 2014. https://higherlogicdownload.s3.amazonaws.com/SVUNET/c9a8d83b-2044-4a4eb3eccd4b2f542939/UploadedImages/Documents/Performance%20Guidelines%202017/Performance%20Guideline%20LE%20Venous.pdf. Accessed December 1, 2017.

Suggested Reading

Grant EC. Upper extremity venous imaging with color flow Doppler. In: Bernstein EF, editor. Vascular diagnosis. St. Louis: Mosby; 1994. p. 944–50.

Grassi CJ, Polak JF. Axillary and subclavian venous thrombosis: follow-up evaluation with color Doppler flow US and venography. Radiology. 1990;175(3):651–4.

Talbot SR, Oliver MA. Techniques of venous imaging. Pasadena: Appleton Davies, Inc; 1992.

Duplex Ultrasound of the Lower Limb: Superficial Venous System

12

Ryan T. Brooks and Anahita Dua

Purpose

The duplex ultrasound examination of the deep and superficial venous systems of the lower extremities is designed to evaluate for:

- Deep vein thrombosis (*DVT*)
- Valvular incompetence within the deep, superficial, and perforating venous systems

R. T. Brooks (✉) · A. Dua
Division of Vascular and Endovascular Surgery, Department of Surgery, Massachusetts General Hospital/Harvard Medical School, Boston, MA, USA
e-mail: rtbrooks@mgh.harvard.edu; adua1@mgh.harvard.edu

C. Echevarria et al. (eds.), *The Massachusetts General Hospital Protocols and Procedures for Venous Disease*,
https://doi.org/10.1007/978-3-032-05708-2_12

This examination is essential for guiding management strategies in chronic venous insufficiency and venous thromboembolic disease.

Clinical Indications

Indications for this study include, but are not limited to:

- Varicose veins
- Leg pain
- Leg swelling or edema
- Postoperative follow-up
- Suspected deep or superficial venous thrombosis
- Non-healing ulcers
- Stasis dermatitis
- Previous diagnosis of deep vein thrombosis

Preparation and Infection Control

Prior to the examination:

- All equipment and hard surfaces must be disinfected using hospital-approved ABI Sani-Cloth wipes.
- Examination tables should be draped with a disposable sheet or washable linen.
- Patients are asked to remove pants and socks and to wear disposable shorts or a washable gown.

Required Equipment

- *Ultrasound Probes*:
  - C1–6 curved array probe
  - L2–9 and L8–18 linear array probes
- *Cuff Inflation Devices*:
  - Pneumatic rapid cuff inflation device
  - Inflation cuff

- *Additional Supplies*:
  - Sterile and non-sterile ultrasound gel
  - Transeptic cleaner
  - Cloth towels
  - Adjustable stool for the sonographer
  - Exam bed or stretcher with height adjustment
  - Step or stand with handle for patient support

Patient History and Positioning

A comprehensive patient history should include presenting symptoms, risk factors, and prior interventions. A brief physical examination should evaluate for:

- Varicosities
- Skin changes
- Reticular veins
- Ulceration
- Sites of previous treatments

Initial Positioning: Supine

- Begin with the patient in a supine position to assess the compressibility of the deep and superficial veins. Document any evidence of thrombus or chronic changes in the deep or superficial system.
- Spectral waveform assessment of bilateral common femoral veins is performed in the supine position to document venous phasicity or lack thereof.

Reflux Assessment: Standing

- Transition the patient to a standing position, supported by a raised examination table.

- The examined leg should be externally rotated, with body weight shifted to the contralateral limb.
- If standing is not tolerated, position the patient in reverse Trendelenburg using a tilt table with footboard.
- Monitor patient for discomfort or signs of vasovagal syncope or nausea. If this occurs, the exam should be paused immediately, and the sonographer should lay the patient down on the bed or ask them to sit. The clinician should provide support as needed (e.g., glass of water, wet cloth, open a window).

Ultrasound Technique

Reflux Assessment

Reflux is evaluated using spectral Doppler with the probe positioned in the longitudinal view only, using the following method:

- A distal augmentation maneuver is performed with a pneumatic inflation device and an inflatable cuff placed on the proximal calf or ankle.
- Inflation pressure should be set at 110 mmHg (pressure can be decreased if the patient reports discomfort).
- The sweep speed of the spectral waveform should be increased to 10–12 s to allow the entire duration of reflux to be documented.
- Valsalva maneuvers are not recommended due to variability in patient effort.
- Reflux is confirmed by a Doppler shift (flow reversal on the spectral waveform from below the baseline to above the baseline) (Fig. 12.1).
- The duration of reflux is measured in seconds using calipers.
- Anterior-to-posterior vessel diameters (intima-to-intima) and vessel depth from the skin surface are recorded throughout the thigh and calf (Fig. 12.2).

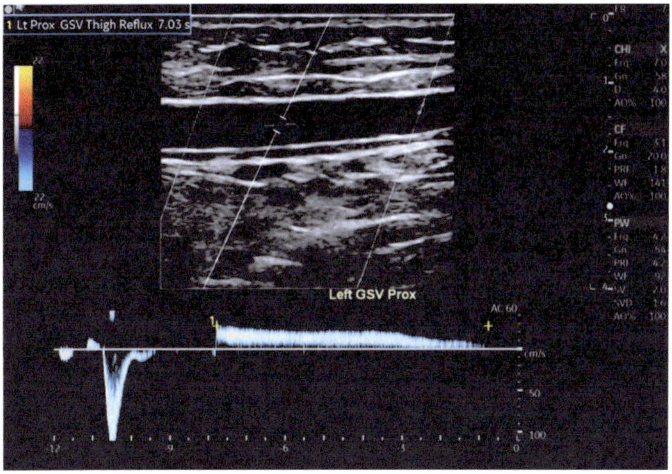

Fig. 12.1 Spectral waveform showing a Doppler shift following a distal augmentation

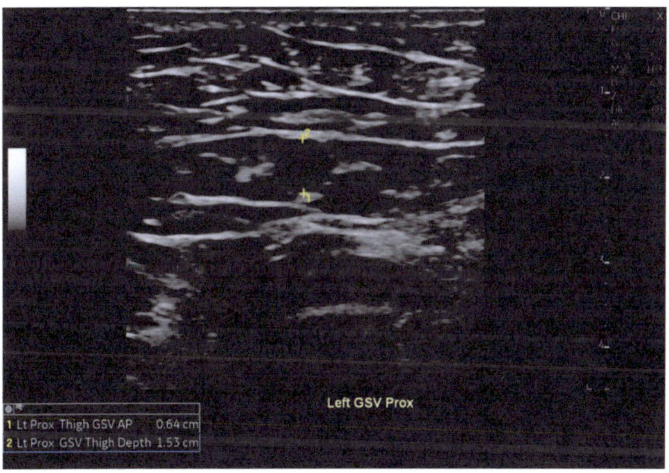

Fig. 12.2 Diameter and depth measurements of the GSV

Examination Protocol

1. *Saphenofemoral Junction (SFJ)*
   - Place inflation cuff on the proximal calf.
   - Measure the diameter of the SFJ in B-mode (transverse plane).
   - Obtain a spectral Doppler waveform with distal augmentation (Fig. 12.3).
2. *Common Femoral Vein (CFV)*`
   - Assess for deep venous reflux using spectral Doppler waveform with distal augmentation.
3. *Great Saphenous Vein (GSV)*
   - Evaluate in longitudinal and transverse planes at:
     - Proximal thigh
     - Mid-thigh
     - Knee
   - Measure diameter and depth in the transverse plane.
   - Obtain spectral Doppler waveforms in the longitudinal plane.

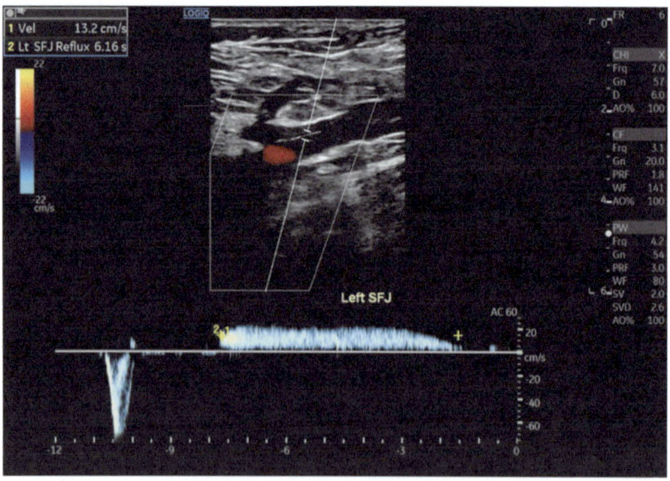

Fig. 12.3 Saphenofemoral junction reflux

4. *Anterior Accessory Saphenous Vein (AASV)*
   - If present, follow its course transversely, obtaining depth and diameter measurements.
   - Assess competence at all thigh levels via spectral Doppler waveforms with distal augmentation.
5. *Tributaries and Perforators*
   - Note anatomical locations, diameter, and depth measurements.
   - Assess for reflux with spectral Doppler waveforms with distal augmentation.
6. *Length of Vessel Within the Fascia*
   - If the GSV, AASV, or SSV are incompetent, measure the distance from the SFJ or SPJ to the point where the vessel exits the fascia (Fig. 12.4).
7. *Mid Femoral Vein*
   - Assess for deep venous reflux using a spectral Doppler waveform with distal augmentation.
8. *Posterior Leg Evaluation*
   - With the patient turned away, assess the following:
     - Popliteal vein
     - Saphenopopliteal junction (SPJ)

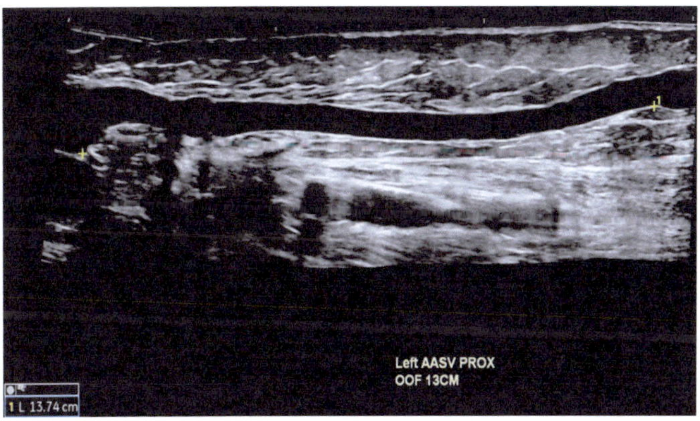

Fig. 12.4 Length of the vessel which remains within the fascia 13 (cm). (Longitudinal View)

  - Small saphenous vein (SSV)
  - Posterior thigh extension vein (PTE)
  - Enlarged perforators
9. *Calf Assessment*
   - Move the cuff to the lower calf/ankle and perform distal augmentation with spectral analysis of the following vessels.
     - SPJ at the popliteal fossa or the PTE in the posterior thigh
     - SSV at proximal and mid-calf levels.
     - GSV at the proximal calf
10. *Perforator Evaluation*
    - Atypical tributaries should be followed proximally to document potential communication with a perforator or a possible pelvic source.
    - If an ulcer is present, the patient should sit on the edge of the bed/stretcher with the leg dangling.
    - Evaluate calf perforators with spectral Doppler and obtain diameter measurements at the fascial border.
    - Reflux can be elicited using distal augmentation at the ankle/foot or by asking the patient to flex the ankle.

Image Acquisition Requirements

Grayscale Compression Imaging

Transverse views with and without compression for:

- CFV/SFJ
- Proximal profunda femoris vein
- Proximal, mid, and distal segments of the femoral vein
- GSV (proximal thigh, mid-thigh, knee, and proximal calf)
- AASV (if visualized)
- Popliteal vein
- Gastrocnemius, posterior tibial, peroneal, and small saphenous veins
- Any additional varicosities demonstrating thrombus

Anterior-Posterior Grayscale with Measurements

Record vessel diameter and depth at:

- SFJ
- GSV (proximal thigh, mid-thigh, knee, and proximal calf)
- AASV
- SPJ (if present)
- SSV
- PTE (if present and incompetent)
- Any incompetent tributaries or perforators

Spectral Doppler Requirements (with Distal Augmentation)

- CFV
- SFJ
- GSV (proximal, mid-thigh, knee, and calf)
- Mid femoral vein
- Popliteal vein
- SSV (at SPJ when visualized)
- AASV
- PTE
- Any incompetent tributaries or perforators

Interpretation Criteria

Vein Type	Reflux Threshold (s)
Superficial veins	>0.5
Deep veins	>1.0
Perforator veins	≥0.35

Phasicity Assessment

- Normal: Symmetrical phasicity between the right and left CFVs
- Abnormal: Monophasic or asymmetric flow
- New findings of monophasic flow in the CFV or external iliac vein should be reported immediately to the clinical team

Incidental Findings

Any incidental anatomic or pathologic findings (e.g., pelvic source veins, collateral formation, occluded arteries, soft tissue masses) must be documented and included in the final report.

Summary

A step-by-step guide to assessing the deep and superficial venous systems for the presence of valvular insufficiency. Using a variety of clinical tools, a sonographer will test multiple segments of the vessels in the lower extremity to identify or rule out venous incompetence. To better assist the provider with a treatment plan, the sonographer is tasked with describing the anatomy and functionality of the superficial venous system.

Suggested Reading

Pieri A, Gatti M, Santini M, Marcelli F, Carnemolla A. Ultrasonographic anatomy of the deep veins of the lower extremity. J Vasc Technol. 2002;26(3):201–11.

Welch HJ, Faliakou EC, McLaughlin RL, Umphrey SE, Belkin M, O'Donnell TF. Comparison of descending phlebography with quantitative photoplethysmography and duplex quantitative valve closure time in assessing deep venous reflux. J Vasc Surg. 1992;16:913–20.

Van Bemmelen PS, Bedford G, Beach K, Strandness DE. Quantitative segmental evaluation of venous reflux with duplex ultrasound scanning. J Vasc Surg. 1989;10:425–31.

Abdominopelvic Venous Duplex Ultrasound

13

Ryan T. Brooks and Anahita Dua

Introduction

Pelvic venous disorders (PeVD) represent a range of hemodynamic abnormalities involving reflux and obstruction in the abdominal and pelvic venous systems. These conditions are underdiagnosed contributors to chronic pelvic pain, varicosities, and venous insufficiency. This chapter outlines a comprehensive duplex ultrasound protocol designed to evaluate pelvic venous anatomy and physiology with diagnostic precision.

R. T. Brooks (✉) · A. Dua
Division of Vascular and Endovascular Surgery, Department of Surgery, Massachusetts General Hospital/Harvard Medical School, Boston, MA, USA
e-mail: rtbrooks@mgh.harvard.edu; adua1@mgh.harvard.edu

C. Echevarria et al. (eds.), *The Massachusetts General Hospital Protocols and Procedures for Venous Disease*,
https://doi.org/10.1007/978-3-032-05708-2_13

Clinical Presentations of Pelvic Venous Disorders

Pelvic venous pathology is commonly associated with one or more of the following clinical syndromes (Meissner et al.):

1. *Left flank pain and hematuria* due to left renal vein (LRV) compression
2. *Chronic pelvic pain* associated with pelvic varicosities
3. *Venous claudication* secondary to iliac vein obstruction
4. *Lower extremity varicosities*, in typical or atypical distributions, often recurrent post-treatment (Meissner et al.)

Indications for Examination

Pelvic venous duplex ultrasound is indicated for patients with:

- Chronic pelvic pain (>6 months)
- Pelvic heaviness
- Dyspareunia
- Dysmenorrhea
- Hemorrhoids
- Vulvar, scrotal, or gluteal varicosities
- Urinary urgency or frequency
- Lumbar or post-coital pain

Patient Preparation and Positioning

- Fasting: 8–12 h prior to examination to limit bowel gas.
- Positioning: Start patient in the supine position with the head of the bed raised 15°–20°.
  - Arms are rested at their side and their head is supported with a pillow; progress to reverse Trendelenburg or standing as indicated.
- Repositioning helps differentiate positional vs. fixed compressions.

⚠ *Ergonomic Note*: Scanning while the patient is standing requires sonographer shoulder abduction; limit scan time in this position.

Equipment and Probes

- Curved linear probe (C1–6)
- Linear probes (L2–9, L8–18)
- Intracavitary probe (IC 5–9)
- Sterile ultrasound gel (internal portion of exam)
- Non-sterile ultrasound gel (external portion of exam)
- Sterile ultrasound probe cover
- Trophon disinfection system

Scanning Technique

The vessels examined are the inferior vena cava (IVC), left renal vein (LRV), bilateral common iliac veins (CIV), bilateral ovarian/gonadal veins, bilateral internal iliac veins (IIV) and associated branches, pelvic adnexa, para uterine veins, scrotal varicoceles, and any potential pelvic escape points.

Limited assessment of the aorta and bilateral common iliac arteries is included to rule out arterial aneurysm, which may be a contributing factor to any venous compression syndrome.

If a patient has a common iliac vein stent, spectral analysis, diameter measurements, and color-assisted Doppler images should be obtained at the proximal, mid, and distal segments of the stent to assess patency. Spectral Doppler waveforms of the ipsilateral profunda femoris vein and common femoral vein should also be assessed to ensure proper venous outflow.

Before performing a transvaginal assessment, the clinic's sterile protocol should be followed. The sterilized intracavitary ultrasound probe is removed from its sleeve and sterile ultrasound gel is placed on the tip of the probe. A sterile probe sleeve is then carefully placed over the entire ultrasound probe and the first 6 inches of the cord. Sterile ultrasound gel is placed on top of the sterile ultrasound probe and the probe is carefully inserted into the vaginal canal by the technologist. If a male sonographer is performing a transvaginal exam, a female clinical staff member is required to be physically present throughout the exam. This method of "chaperoning" may also be advised for a female technologist performing a scrotal exam on a male patient.

Once the transvaginal assessment is complete, the technologist will go through the probe sterilization protocol utilizing vendor approved sanitizing/drying wipes, before placing the probe in the Trophon sterilizing unit. Once the probe has been properly sterilized, it is to be placed in a clinic approved probe cover/sleeve and stored in an assigned cabinet.

Protocol Overview

Inferior Vena Cava (IVC)

- Assess for duplication, hypoplasia, filter, thrombosis.
- Transverse B-mode and longitudinal Doppler (proximal, mid, distal)
- Key landmarks: xiphoid to umbilicus

Common Iliac Veins (CIV)

The iliac veins are initially imaged to assess patency and rule out obstruction, in the form of acute or chronic thrombus. The common iliac veins (CIV) are then assessed to detect compression, in the form of diameter reduction, and any changes in peak venous velocity or venous phasicity.

- Use the curved linear probe to evaluate the CIV for patency, compression, and peak venous velocity.
- Measure A/P diameters, proximal to distal, in the longitudinal plane.

  - The diameter of the proximal CIV should be measured at the greatest point of compression (Fig. 13.1a).
  - The distal CIV is to be measured just proximal to the ostium of the internal iliac vein (IIV) (Fig. 13.1b).
- Spectral Doppler waveforms, with peak venous velocity measurements, should be obtained in the longitudinal plane, proximally and distally (Fig. 13.1c, d).
  - The Doppler angle should be set at 60° or lower.
- If the CIV demonstrates a significant diameter reduction or velocity discrepancy in the supine position, rescan the patient in the reverse Trendelenburg position. Note any changes in diameter and velocity ratios in the final report.
- Key landmarks: aorta bifurcation (point of greatest compression of the left CIV), ostium of the internal iliac vein.

Diagnostic Criteria for Common Iliac Vein Compression

- Common Iliac Vein Peak Venous Velocity Ratio
  - CIV velocity (cm/sec. at site of compression)/peripheral CIV velocity.
  - Peak venous velocity ratio of ≥2.5 is considered diagnostically significant.
    - Monophasic waveforms (Fig. 13.1e), peak venous flow (<5 cm/s), or absence of flow are all significant findings and should be noted in the final report.
- Common Iliac Vein Diameter Ratio
  - Peripheral CIV (mm)/central CIV (site of greatest compression).
  - Diameter reduction of ≥50% is considered diagnostically significant.
    - Vessel wall thickening or evidence of synechiae within the lumen of the vein are significant findings and should be noted in the final report.

In the scenario where the velocity ratios or diameter reduction thresholds have not been met, yet there is evidence of some level of compression, the ultrasound report should note that the ratios are elevated.

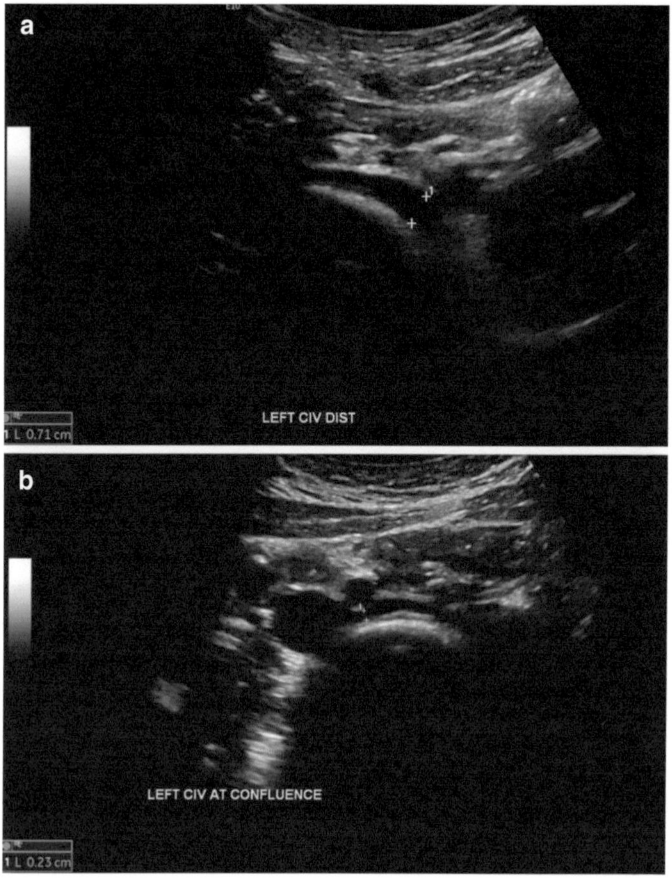

Fig. 13.1 (**a**) Distal Common Iliac vein diamter 7.1 mm. (**b**) Proximal Common Iliac vein diameter of 2.3 mm. Diameter Ratio of 3.08 (Distal CIV 7.1 mm/Proximal CIV 2.3 mm). >50% reduction in vessel diameter. (**c**) Peak venous velocity of the left Common iliac vein at site of greatest compression. (**d**) Common Iliac Vein Peak Venous Velocity Ratio 2.57 (Proximal CIV 67.8/ Distal CIV 26 cm/s). Diameter reduction of ≥50% and a peak venous velocity ratio of ≥2.5 is considered diagnostically significant. (**e**) Monophasic venous flow profile. (**f**) Right Internal Iliac Vein

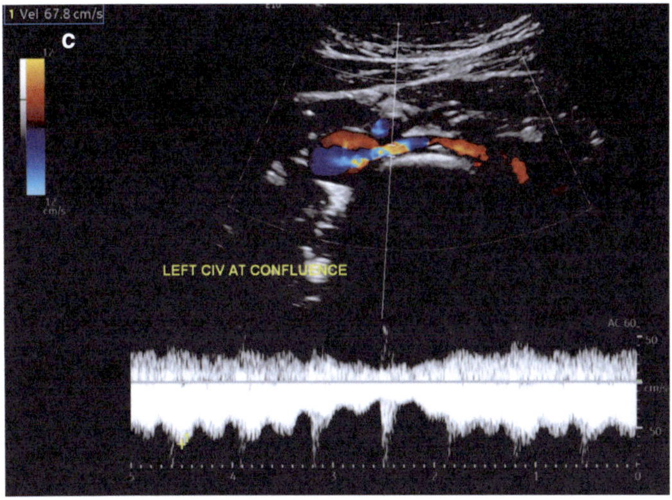

Fig. 13.1 (continued)

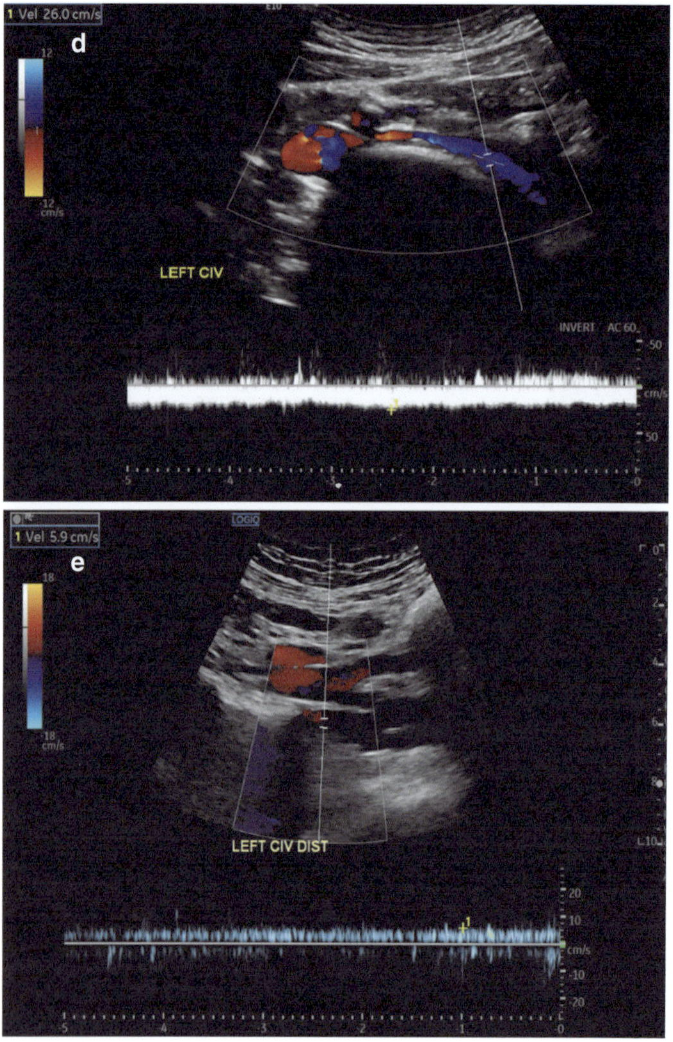

Fig. 13.1 (continued)

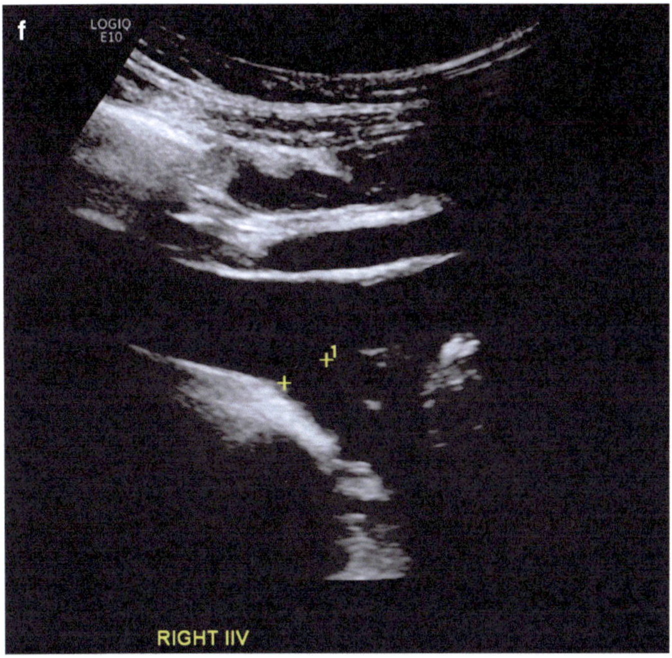

Fig. 13.1 (continued)

Common Iliac Vein Stent Assessment

After a CIV stent has been placed, patency of the stent and inflow/outflow vessels are assessed via duplex ultrasound. Stent surveillance is performed 1 month after initial placement, and then every 3–4 months for the first 2 years. Depending on the patient's symptoms and circumstances, assessment of stent patency is typically performed every 1–2 years.

In the setting of a common iliac vein stent, assess the IVC (outflow), entirety of the stent (proximal, mid, distal), and inflow vein (EIV/CFV).

- Perform spectral analysis with the Doppler angle set at 60° or lower.
- Diameter measurements at each segment of the stent.
- Grayscale and color-assisted Doppler still images should be obtained at the proximal, mid, and distal segments of the stent to assess for patency and color-filling defect.
- Spectral Doppler waveforms of the ipsilateral profunda femoris vein and common femoral vein should also be assessed to ensure proper venous inflow to the stent.

Internal Iliac Veins (IIV)

- Use both transabdominal and transvaginal views.
- Document reflux via controlled Valsalva maneuvers.
  - Retrograde flow during Valsalva maneuver is diagnostically significant.
  - The duration of reflux should be recorded with calipers.
  - Increase spectral sweep speed ≥8 s.

The internal iliac veins (IIV) are imaged using the curved linear probe as well as with the intracavitary/transvaginal probe.

Using the curved linear probe transabdominally, the ostium of the internal iliac veins is located just caudal to the distal segment of the common iliac vein (Fig. 13.1f).

- Measure the diameter of this vessel and ask the patient to perform a controlled Valsalva maneuver to elicit venous reflux.

Before performing the transvaginal assessment, follow the sterile protocol (see section "Scanning Technique").

- When assessing the internal iliac veins using the transvaginal probe, the vessels can be located on the lateral walls of the pelvis posterior to the ovaries. A/P diameter measurements are obtained at mid-vein followed by spectral Doppler assessment to rule out venous reflux. The patient is asked to again perform a controlled Valsalva maneuver during the pulsed-wave Doppler assessment. Absence of flow during the Valsalva maneuver is a normal finding. The vessel is refluxing when turbulent flow is present during the Valsalva maneuver.

Left Renal Vein (LRV)

The LRV is examined throughout its course to document obstruction or compression. The primary cause of renal vein compression occurs where the LRV crosses superior to the abdominal aorta and inferior to the superior mesenteric artery (SMA). The extrinsic compression of the surrounding arteries can cause the left renal vein to narrow drastically; this is often referred to as anterior nutcracker syndrome.

Although not as common, the LRV may also course retroaortic, and extrinsic compression may occur as the vein courses between the abdominal aorta and the thoracic vertebrae (Fig. 13.2a) (posterior nutcracker anatomy).

Imaging the LRV

The LRV crosses the abdomen, left to right, ultimately draining directly into the IVC. The LRV can be identified by imaging the IVC and aorta in the transverse plane. Starting at the xiphoid process, slowly sweep proximal to distal to locate the SMA (the second branch of the abdominal aorta). Once the SMA is identified, the LRV will typically cross the abdomen and course just posterior to the SMA. Light probe pressure should be utilized during assessment so as not to artificially compress the vein. Due to the anatomic position, the LRV will be visualized longitudinally while the probe is in a transverse orientation. In this longitudinal view, AP diameters are obtained at the narrowest point of the LRV (Fig. 13.2b). The probe is then positioned toward the left kidney and the diameter of the distal segment of the LRV will be documented (Fig. 13.2c).

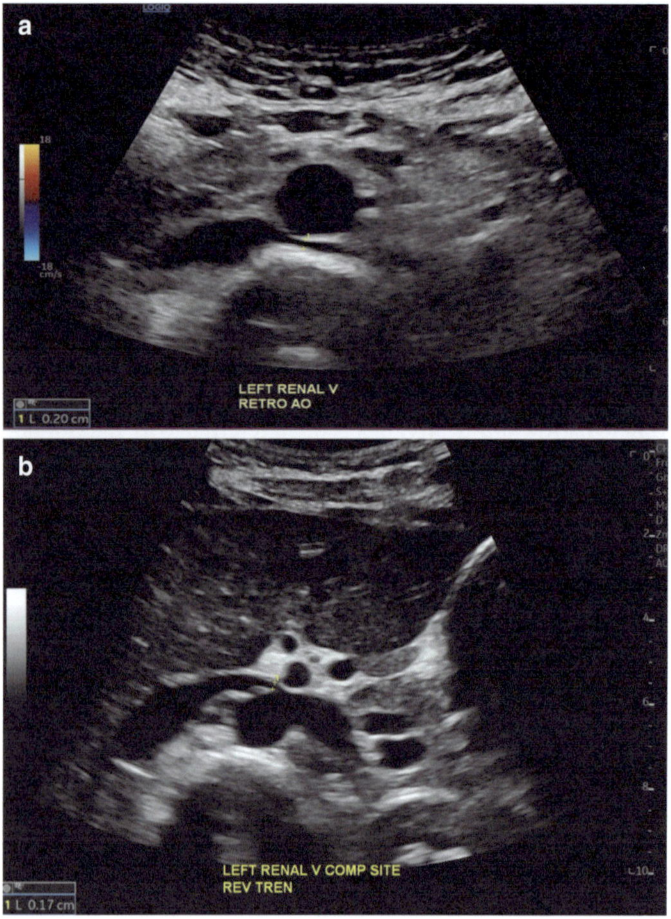

Fig. 13.2 (**a**) Retro-Aortic Renal Vein. (**b**) Left Renal vein diameter at site of greatest compression. (**c**) LRV Diameter Ratio 7.6 (Distal Renal vein 13 mm/ Renal vein @ site of compression 1.7 mm) (Diameter ratio >5.0 is consistent with renal vein compression anatomy). (**d**) Left Renal vein peak venous velocity at the site of greatest compression. (**e**) LRV Peak Venous Velocity Ratio 6.9 (LRV @ site of compression 88.1/LRV Distal 12.6 cm/s) (Peak Venous Velocity ratio >5.0 is consistent with Left renal vein compression anatomy). (**f**) Grayscale image of the left ovarian vein functioning as a direct outflow pathway for the left renal vein. (**g**) Color Doppler image of the left ovarian vein functioning as a direct outflow pathway for the left renal vein

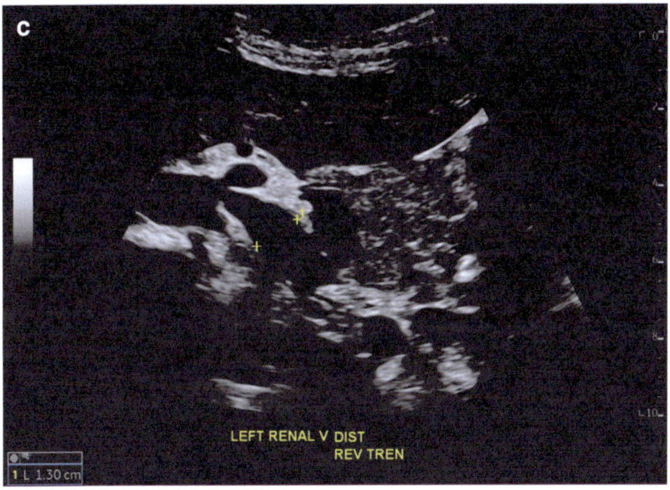

Fig. 13.2 (continued)

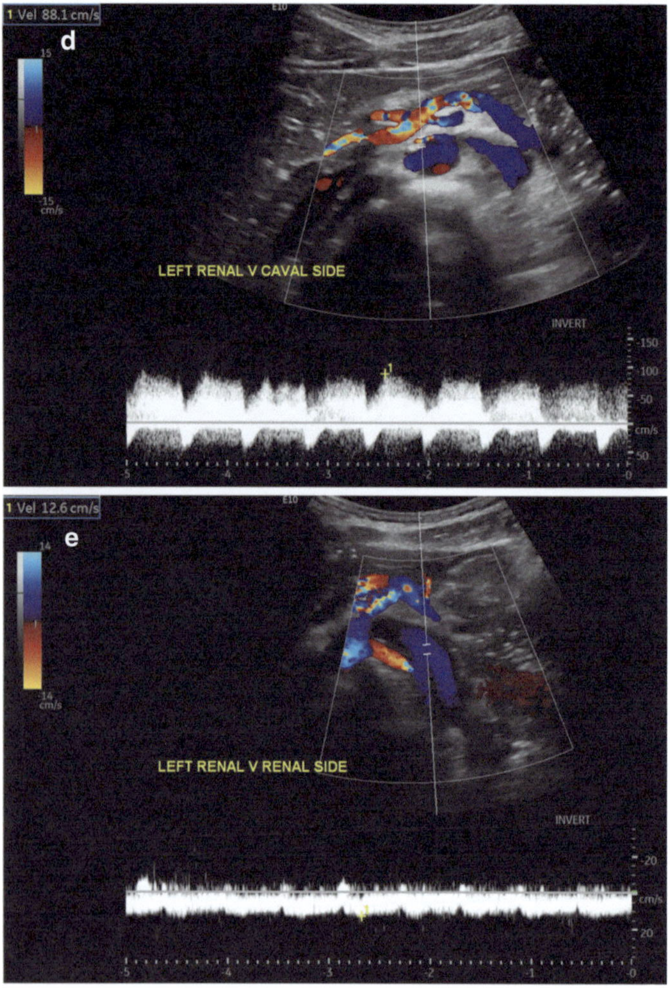

Fig. 13.2 (continued)

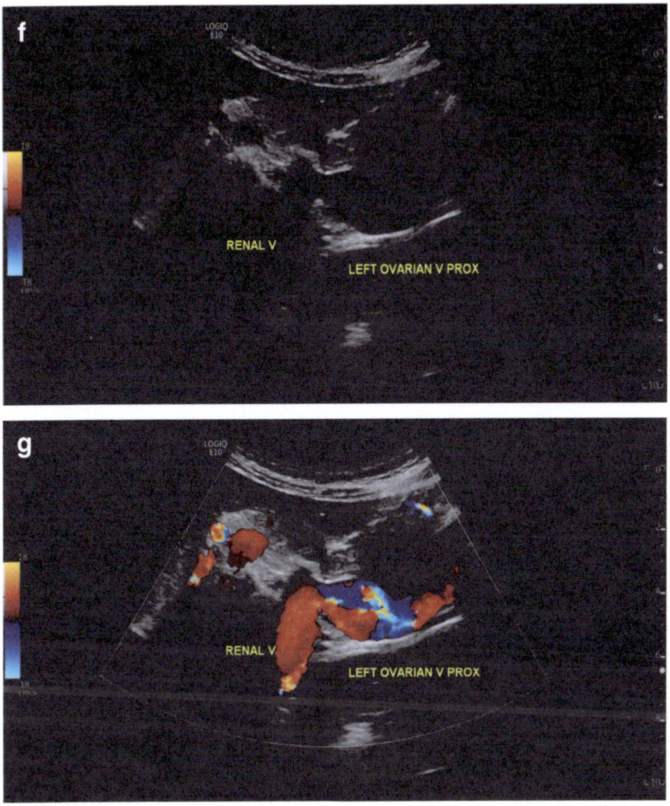

Fig. 13.2 (continued)

In conjunction with A/P measurements, spectral Doppler assessment of peak venous velocities in the above-mentioned locations is performed using a Doppler angle of incidence of 60° or less, (Fig. 13.2d, e).

The right renal vein is examined rarely. Spectral assessment is only performed if the right ovarian vein communicates with the right renal vein instead of the IVC.

Diagnostic Criteria for Renal Vein Compression

- Establish if the patient has anterior nutcracker anatomy (LRV between SMA and aorta) or posterior nutcracker syndrome (LRV between aorta and vertebrae)
- Measure LRV diameters and velocities at:
  - Point of greatest compression
  - Distal to compression (peripheral LRV)
  - Calculate compression and diameter ratios

LRV Peak Velocity Ratio (velocity of greatest compression/velocity of distal renal vein).

Peak venous velocity ratio >5.0 is consistent with renal vein compression anatomy.

LRV Diameter Ratio (distal renal vein/renal vein @ greatest site of compression).

Diameter ratio >5.0 is consistent with renal vein compression anatomy.

Significant findings of the LRV which should be included in the report: elevated velocity/diameter ratios, diminished or absent of flow in the LRV, presence of collateral veins, and flow from diversion for the LRV to the left ovarian/gonadal vein.

If the LRV compression is significant, there may not be any flow to sample at the confluence of the SMA. In this scenario, the LRV compression may be so severe that spontaneous reflux is documented within the LOV with the patient in the supine position (Fig. 13.2f, g). The continuous flow would suggest a downstream reservoir of collateral vessels within the pelvic cavity, resulting in adnexal and para-uterine varicosities.

Ovarian/Gonadal Veins

The ovarian/gonadal veins are examined to detect insufficiency, duplication, thrombus, dilation, and tortuosity.

The left ovarian vein (LOV) is found to the left side of the patient's aorta, at mid-abdomen level, just anterior to the patient's left psoas muscle. The vessel can be identified in the longitudinal and/or transverse planes. Once the LOV is located, it is followed upward to visualize its communication with the LRV. Moving toward the pelvis, one may encounter multiple trunks or ovarian vein tortuosity (Fig. 13.3a, b). A/P diameters, in either transverse or longitudinal planes, of the LOV are obtained distal to its communication with the LRV and just proximal to its communication with the ovary (Fig. 13.3c).

Spectral Doppler waveforms demonstrating direction of flow within the LOV should be documented with the patient in the supine position as well as with the patient in the reverse Trendelenburg or standing positions. Saved images should be annotated with the method in which the waveform was obtained, e.g., LOV (Supine), LOV (Rev-Tren), and LOV (Standing) (Fig. 13.3d). Although Valsalva and distal augmentation maneuvers may elicit reflux, it can be difficult to accurately sample the flow during these maneuvers. The method by which reflux is elicited will help to determine if the reflux is primary or secondary (see diagnostic criteria included).

The right ovarian vein (ROV) is found just above and to the right of the umbilicus on the anterior aspect of the patient's right psoas muscle. Once the ROV is located, you will follow it upward to visualize its communication with the IVC. The ROV will be assessed in the same manner as the LOV.

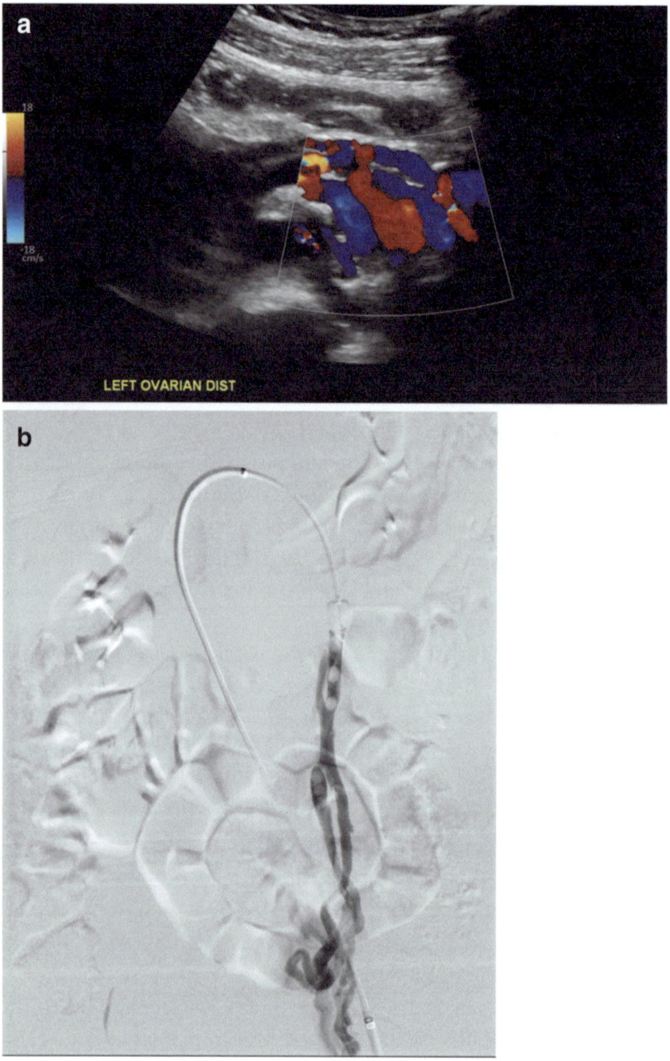

Fig. 13.3 (**a**) Distal Ovarian vein with severe tortuosity, (via Duplex Ultrasound). (**b**) Left Ovarian vein with severe tortuosity as seen with fluoroscopic guidance. (**c**) Dilated Left Ovarian Vein. (**d**) Left Ovarian vein demonstrating retrograde flow in the Reverse Trendelenburg position

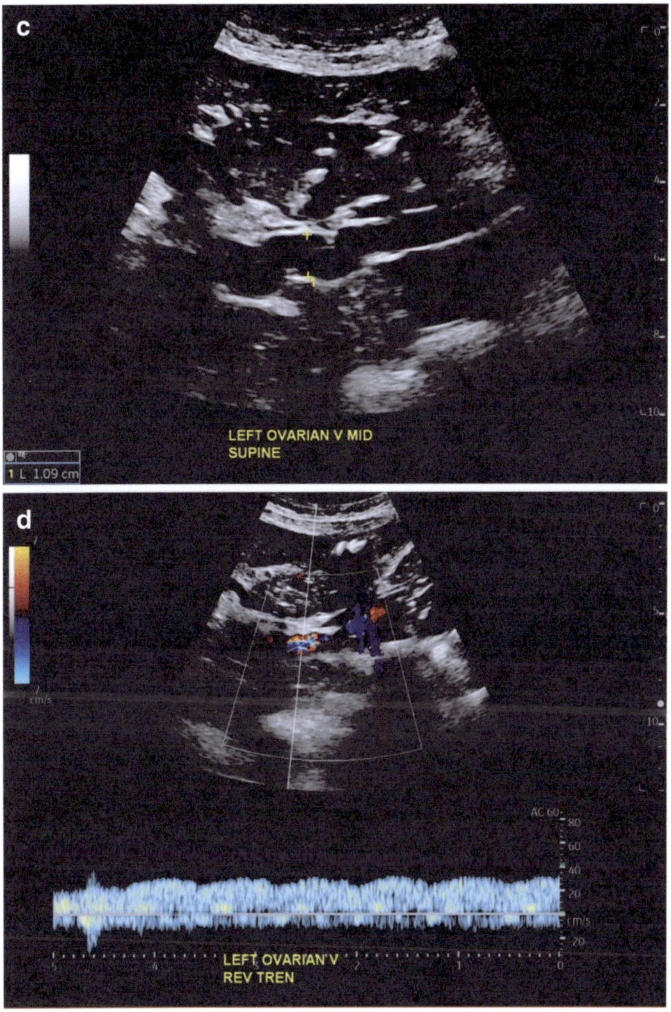

Fig. 13.3 (continued)

Diagnostic Criteria for Ovarian/Gonadal Vein Insufficiency

Any ovarian/gonadal vein with a diameter of ≥6 mm should be considered insufficient.

Reflux in the gonadal veins elicited by Valsalva maneuvers can be difficult to capture due to abdominal motion.

Retrograde flow in the LOV with the patient in the supine or dependent position (Supine, Rev-Tren, or Standing), is a positive finding of venous incompetence. If retrograde flow is present, the following should be considered:

- Spontaneous and continuous reflux in the LOV may indicate a proximal LRV compression.
- Intermittent reflux (lasting >0.5 s) signifies isolated LOV incompetence and can be documented by having the patient perform a controlled Valsalva.

Gonadal/Ovarian Vein Insufficiency

Imaging Protocol

- Identify left ovarian vein (LOV)/right ovarian vein (ROV) and trace from renal origin to pelvic insertion.
- Assess the following parameters:
  - *Diameter*
  - *Tortuosity*
  - *Flow direction (retrograde/antegrade)*
  - *Presence and cause of reflux*

Reflux Evaluation

- Evaluate for reflux in the supine position and during positional changes (Reverse Trendelenburg/Standing).
- Retrograde flow in the LOV with the patient in the supine or dependent position (Supine, Rev-Tren, or Standing), is a positive finding of venous incompetence.
- Determine if reflux is:

- Spontaneous continuous flow in supine or dependent position → *suggests secondary to renal vein compression.*
- Intermittent reflux >0.5 s → *suggests primary venous insufficiency.*

Peri- and Trans-uterine Plexus Veins

Transabdominal Evaluation

The veins within the bilateral pelvic adnexa, as well as any para-uterine veins, are examined for AP diameters, tortuosity, and reflux with controlled Valsalva maneuvers. Dilated peri-uterine veins are identified transabdominally by angling the curved linear probe to the far right or left of the pelvis in a longitudinal plane and slowly scanning from one side of the pelvis across the midline to the opposite side of the pelvis (Fig. 13.4a).

Transvaginal Evaluation

The transvaginal exam begins by following the sterile protocol (see section "Scanning Technique"). Upon insertion of the probe, begin with a coronal and longitudinal cine loop sweep of the uterus.

Pelvic Adnexa

Angle the probe toward the lateral aspects of the uterus to document the presence of ovarian and adnexal varices (Fig. 13.4b). Controlled Valsalva maneuvers are used to document Doppler shifts within the pelvic adnexa. The diameter of any adnexal varices should be measured anterior to posterior.

Internal Iliac Veins

Begin by angling the probe posterolateral to the sidewall of the pelvis.

Utilize color Doppler and spectral analysis to identify adnexal varices communicating with the IIV. Place the spectral Doppler within the lumen of the IIV and ask the patient to perform a controlled Valsalva maneuver.

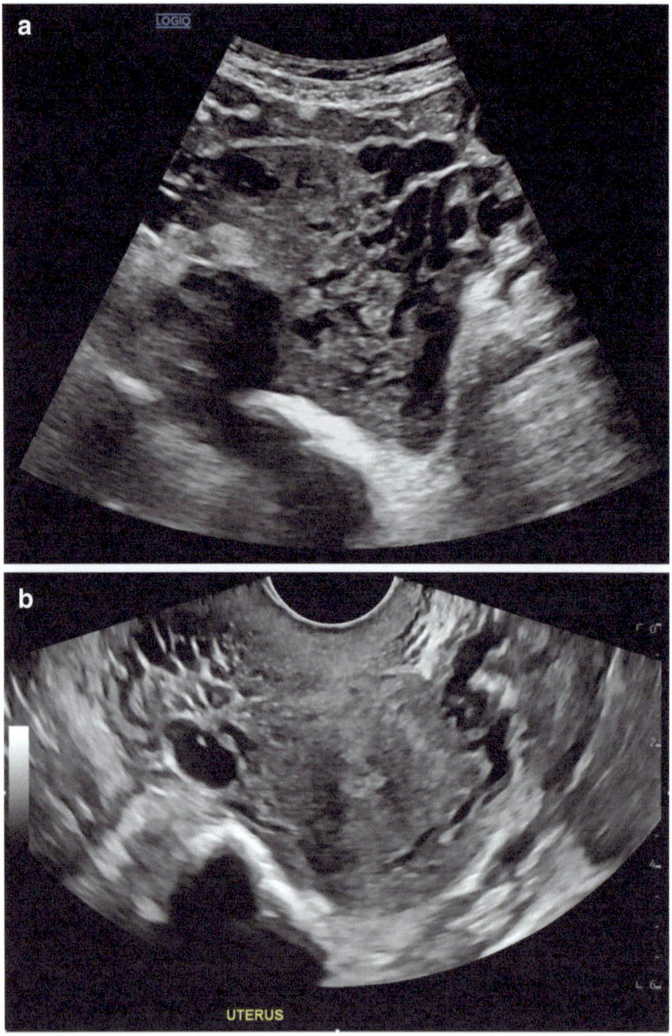

Fig. 13.4 (**a**) Transabdominal vein of a Uterus with left sided adnexal varicosities. (**b**) Transvaginal view of the Uterus with bilateral adnexal varicosities

Peri-anal/Peri-urethral Veins

In the transverse approach, angle the probe posteriorly to evaluate for peri-anal varices. The probe is then angled anteriorly to evaluate any peri-urethral varices. Controlled Valsalva maneuvers are used to induce reflux.

Any incidental findings of ovarian cysts or enlarged uterine fibroids should be documented.

Diagnostic Criteria for Peri and Trans-uterine Plexus Vein Insufficiency

Diameter measurements ≥6 mm, and presence of reflux >0.5 s throughout the Valsalva maneuver is considered diagnostically significant.

Scrotal Varicosities

Assessment of the scrotum should be performed using a high-frequency linear transducer with the patient in the standing position. A/P diameter measurements of the largest varicosity are obtained (Fig. 13.5a), and the patient is asked to perform controlled Valsalva maneuvers. Continuous flow at rest (Fig. 13.5b), or the presence of flow throughout the Valsalva maneuver, (>0.5 s), is considered diagnostically significant. Documentation of this finding can be accomplished by recording a cine loop using color Doppler and by measuring the duration of reflux in the spectral waveform.

Pelvic Escape Points

Most patients experiencing pelvic source varicosities should also have a formal lower extremity venous reflux assessment. This exam is typically performed with the patient in a dependent standing position using spectral Doppler analysis in response to inter-

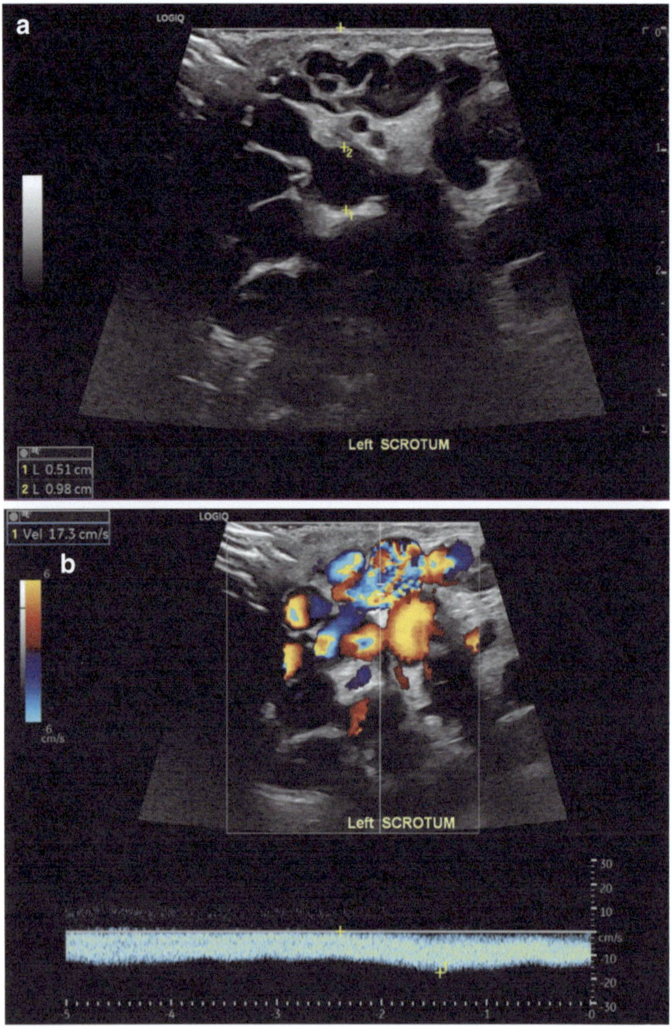

Fig. 13.5 (**a**) Left Scrotal Varicocele. (**b**) Left Scrotal Varicocele demonstrating continuous flow

mittent inflation of a pneumatic compression device. While standing, the hydrostatic pressure will increase visualization of the refluxing varicosities. Using a high-frequency linear probe, the saphenofemoral junction (SFJ) is assessed for competency. The probe is then moved proximal to the SFJ to examine any connection of the pelvic floor varicosities with the lower extremities. Reflux is elicited using a controlled Valsalva maneuver or with the pneumatic cuff inflation device. These vessels tend to be tortuous, and they do not always communicate with the SFJ, GSV, or PTE. They typically remain superficial as they course down the anterior or posterior aspect of the thigh and calf.

Common escape points to be assessed are as follows:

- The *pudendal escape points* often present on the labia or vulva. They communicate with the external pudendal vein, which is a branch of the internal iliac vein. They can be located by moving the probe medially to the perineum.
  - Asking the patient to perform a controlled Valsalva maneuver should illicit continuous flow.
- The *inguinal escape point* (round ligament vein) can be found by tracing an existing varicosity to the inguinal canal.
- The *obturator/gluteal escape point* can be found by following veins in the posterior thigh to the gluteal area to demonstrate connections, via perforators, deeper to the gluteal fascia.

Diagnostic Criteria for Pelvic Escape Points

Reflux with controlled Valsalva, or distal augmentation lasting $>$0.5 s.

Summary Checklist

Structure	Assessments
IVC	Patency, thrombus, duplication
CIV/EIV	Compression ratios, diameter ratios, obstruction
IIV	Diameter, direction of flow, reflux with Valsalva
LRV	Compression ratios, diameter ratios, absence of flow, retro-aortic

Structure	Assessments
Gonadal veins	Diameter, tortuosity, direction of flow (retrograde/antegrade)
Uterine plexus	Diameter, reflux with Valsalva
Escape points	Reflux mapping to SFJ, GSV, or PTE

Summary

Duplex ultrasound of the abdominal and pelvic veins is a safe, non-invasive, and highly accurate imaging modality used to assess for venous compression syndromes. This technique enables real-time evaluation of venous blood velocity, vessel diameter, and the direction of flow. By performing the examination in multiple patient positions—including supine, reverse Trendelenburg, and standing—sonographers can document hemodynamic changes that may suggest positional or anatomical venous compression.

This protocol is designed to guide sonographers through the anatomical landmarks necessary for a comprehensive assessment of the iliac, renal, and gonadal venous systems. Careful adherence to these guidelines supports accurate diagnosis and aids in the detection of clinically significant venous abnormalities.

References

1. Meissner MH, Khilnani NM, et al. The symptoms-varices-pathophysiology classification of pelvic venous disorders. J Vasc Surg Venous Lymphat Disord. 2021;9(3):568–84.

Suggested Reading

Labropoulos N, Jasinski PT, et al. A standardized ultrasound approach to pelvic congestion syndrome. Phlebology. 2017;32(9):608–19.

Metzger PB, Rossi FH, et al. Criteria for detecting significant chronic iliac venous obstructions with duplex ultrasound. J Vasc Surg Venous Lymphat Disord. 2016;4(1):18–27.

Lymphedema: Protocol of Care

14

Carlos Echevarria, Cheryl L. Brunelle,
and Julianne Stoughton

Evaluation

Medical History

Document any previous occurrences of cellulitis, deep vein thrombosis (DVT), trauma, surgeries, or malignancies.

C. Echevarria
Division of Vascular and Endovascular Surgery, Department of Surgery, Massachusetts General Hospital/Harvard Venous & Lymphatic Medicine Alumni, Boston, MA, USA

Division of Vascular and Endovenous Interventions, Veins & Vascular Centers of Excellence, Phoenix, AZ, USA
e-mail: carlos.echevarria@vascular.md

C. L. Brunelle
Department of Physical and Occupational Therapy, Massachusetts General Hospital, Boston, MA, USA
e-mail: cbrunelle@mgh.harvard.edu

J. Stoughton (✉)
Division of Vascular and Endovascular Surgery, Department of Surgery, Massachusetts General Hospital/Harvard Medical School, Boston, MA, USA
e-mail: jstoughton@mgh.harvard.edu

C. Echevarria et al. (eds.), *The Massachusetts General Hospital Protocols and Procedures for Venous Disease*,
https://doi.org/10.1007/978-3-032-05708-2_14

Social History

Assess the patient's prior level of functionality and include any relevant travel history.

Medications

Review the patient's current medications that could potentially affect fluid balance (e.g., CCB).

Examination (The *AFTD-Pitting Test)*

*A*natomical location of edema, *F*orce required to pit, *T*ime (quantified), *D*efinition of edema.

Stemmer's sign (a negative Stemmer's sign has a poor negative predictive value, especially in patients with normal BMI).

Limb Girth in Supine Position and Perometer Measures

For upper extremity measurements, mark the skin every 5 cm starting at the proximal tip of the ulnar styloid process. For lower extremity measurements, mark the skin every 10 cm starting at the lateral malleolus.

Grades or Stages of Lymphedema (ISL Consensus)

Stage 0: Impaired lymphatic transport (as illustrated by lymphoscintigraphy) in the absence of swelling or with subtle signs and symptoms

Stage I: Pitting edema, partially reversible with elevation

Stage II: Non-pitting edema, brawny skin, not reversible with elevation

Stage III: Lymphostatic elephantitis, enormous swelling of the involved extremity, fibrosis and hardening of the dermal tissues. Skin papillomas, acanthosis, fat deposits, and warty overgrowths may be present.

Risk Factors

Chronic venous insufficiency (CVI)
Cancer-related therapy (surgeries or radiation)
Infections (cellulitis)
Extensive thoraxic or pelvic surgeries
Obesity

Differential Diagnosis

- Rule out premenstrual edema, pregnancy, or pre-eclampsia
- Venous disease
- Medication-induced edema
- Obesity
- Lipedema
- Myxedema
- Congestive heart failure
- Pulmonary hypertension
- Protein-losing pathologies (hepatic, renal, or enteropathies)

Imaging Studies

Lymphoscintigraphy

Radionuclide lymphoscintigraphy is the gold standard for diagnosing lymphedema, serving as a confirmatory test in early stages or for surgical planning in advanced cases.

Injection: Technetium-99 (Tc-99) radiotracer
Imaging technology: Gamma camera

Indicators of lymphatic dysfunction:

Delayed or asymmetric lymph node visualization, absent lymphatic channels, collateral pathways, interrupted vessels, deep system visualization, or dermal backflow

Near-Infrared Contrast Lymphography

ICG lymphography is used preoperatively to identify functional lymphatic channels and guide surgical incision placement. Additionally, it can confirm the patency of lymphatic vessels immediately after surgical anastomosis.

Injection: Indocyanine green (ICG) dye

Imaging technology: Infrared camera

Indicators of lymphatic dysfunction:

Linear patterns indicate normally functioning lymphatic channels (may be observed in patients with mild lymphedema symptoms). Dermal backflow patterns, which are nonlinear and indicate abnormal lymphatic fluid movement, are associated with more severe cases of lymphedema.

Magnetic Resonance Lymphography

Mostly used for the evaluation of central conducting lymphatics and alternate lymphatic pathways such as thoracic duct pathologies, lymphatic leaks, and other lymphatic abnormalities. It has been used to detail the lymphatic system, which is essential for planning surgical interventions such as lymphaticovenous anastomosis (LVA) or vascularized lymph node transfer (VLNT).

Injection: Gadolinium-based

Imaging technology: Magnetic resonance

Indicators of lymphatic dysfunction:

Evaluates abnormal lymphatic vessel morphology (dilation, tortuosity, hypoplasia, hyperplasia), lymph node abnormalities, contrast agent distribution (delayed uptake, stasis, pooling or stagnation, extravasation), collateral pathways (dermal backflow, collateral vessels), edema (high signal intensity), fibrosis (low signal intensity).

Diagnosis

Clinical examination is sufficient for the diagnosis of lymphedema. A 2.0 cm difference between the affected and unaffected limb is considered clinically significant and a sign of lymphedema (Fig. 14.1). All patients with CEAP C3-C6 should be considered as phlebo-lymphedema patients.

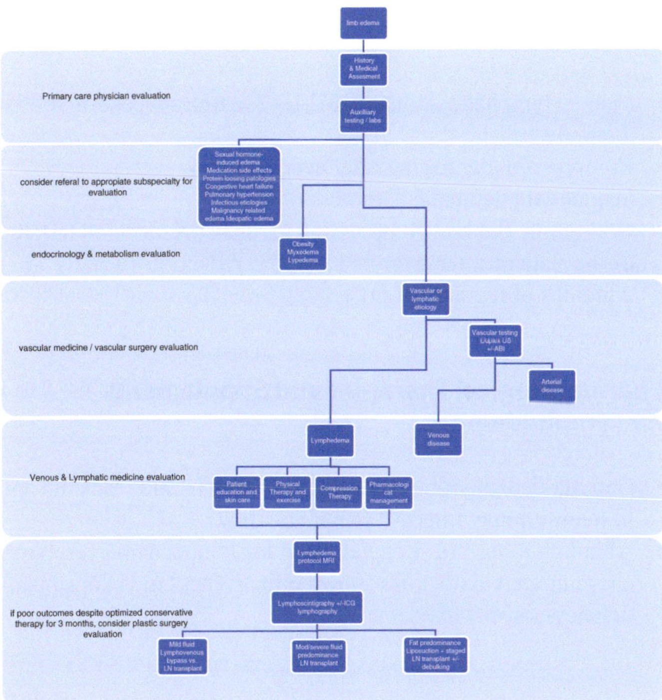

Fig. 14.1 Title: Organizational chart for the management of limb edema

Medical Management

Patient Education

- 1–3% volume reduction occurs after 1–5 h of elevation
- Home program for exercises, self-massage, compression wrapping
- Skin care

Physical Therapy Training

- Therapeutic exercise program including ROM, stretching, and strengthening
- Soft tissue mobilization/myofascial release

Compression

- Manual lymphatic drainage (MLD) 2–3 times/week for at least 3 months
- Compression bandaging after every session
- Sequential pneumatic compression daily
- Non-elastic flat knit compression garment prescription tailored to the patient after maximal volume reduction (usually after 2 months of regular MLD)

Pharmacological Therapies and Supplements for Lymphedema

- Gamma-benzopyrones (flavonoids, which include diosmin and hesperidin) may improve lymphatic flow
- Although it has not been validated for lymphedema yet, horse chestnut seed extract has shown effectiveness in venous insufficiency-associated edema

- Lymphedema may develop as a chronic stage of lymphatic filariasis. By that time, parasitic treatment is futile (if acute infection is suspected, night peripheral smear or serologic testing is warranted before treatment with diethylcarbamazine—contact CDC).

Pharmacological Management of Infection in Lymphedema

- Due to the high risk of commensal skin pathogens, including those in the perineal region, consider wide-spectrum antibiotic therapy for at least 7 days
- Low-dose (benzathine) penicillin may be prescribed to decrease chronicity and recurrence of dermatolymphangioadenitis

Other Therapies

- Medical taping
- Aquatic therapy

Surgical Management

Physiologic Procedures

- Lymphovenous Anastomosis/Bypass (LVA)
  Patients with International Society of Lymphedema (ISL) stage I or II lymphedema, compliant with conservative measures, and BMI <30
- Vascularized Lymph Node Transfer (VLNT)
  Patients with ISL stage II lymphedema with dysfunctional native lymph nodes, dermal backflow, and lymphatic channels not amenable for LVA.

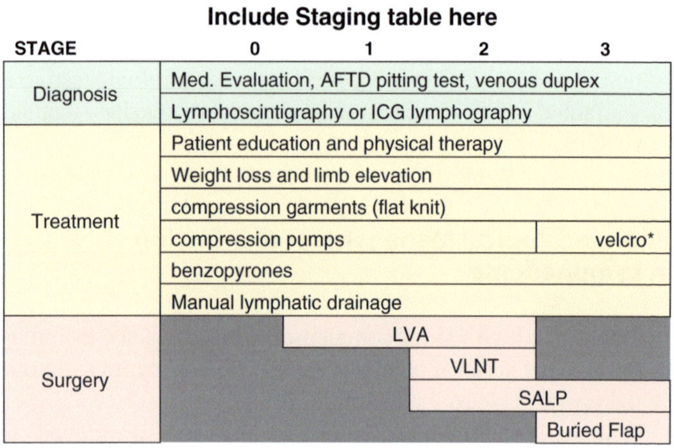

Fig. 14.2 Lymphedema management based on staging

Ablative Procedures

- Liposuction or Suction-Assisted Protein Lipectomy (SALP) ISL stages II or III who have failed compression therapy and have recurrent episodes of cellulitis. The goal is to reduce the solid hypertrophic component of the subcutaneous adipose tissue.
- Buried Flap Procedure
  Debulking surgery removes all skin and soft tissue above the deep fascia. Because of the extensive scarring and other long-term complications, this procedure is typically reserved for the most severe and advanced cases (Fig. 14.2).

MGH Lymphedema Protocol of Care

Multi-Disciplinary Clinical Protocol for Patients with Suspected Lymphedema

Initial Workup

- History and physical exam with AFTD pitting test and photographs
- Height and weight; calculate BMI

- Anthropometrics: circumferences of upper arms, upper and lower legs, and abdomen
- Labs: protein/albumin, liver/renal panel, UA, BNP, HbA1c, fasting glucose, insulin, and lipids; TFTs (if not recently done by PCP)
- Venous Duplex Reflux Exam
  - → referral to venous specialist/interventionalist if venous reflux or obstruction
- Lymphoscintigraphy or Indocyanine Green (ICG) lymphography if no venous disease
  - → referral to Mass General VLM if lymphedema present
  - → referral to Mass General Lipid and Metabolism if lipedema suspected
  - → referral/co-management with MGH Oncology if malignancy present
- *Optional enrollment in Stanford Lymphatic Disease Patient Registry Biorepository*
- *Optional enrollment in MGH Lipid and Metabolic Disorders Biorepository*

Treatment/Monitoring

- Lifestyle Optimization
  - Weight loss and Exercise including water-based (total body compression)
- Therapeutic Options
  - Check for offending medications (calcium channel blockers, beta blockers, glucocorticoids, sex hormones, minoxidil, NSAIDS, clonidine, hydralazine, gabapentin, methyldopa, furosemide, HCTZ)
  - Consider Benzopyrones (hesperidin)/Diosmin—lymphagogues
  - Consider Phentermine—stimulates lipolysis
  - Consider pentoxifilline, statins
  - Consider Metformin—reduces fibrosis
- Referral to Venous & Lymphatic Medicine (VLM) Clinic

  - Compression garments (Class I 20–30 mmHg; circular knit for those with less concomitant lymphedema and upgrade as tolerated; flat knit for edema control)
  - Pneumatic compression devices—E0652 device recommended (segmented, multi-ported pump to allow for individual pressure calibration at each port based on pain and tissue shape); pump garments should wrap around abdomen and pelvis when legs are pumped, and chest when arms are pumped, to avoid accumulation of fluid in these areas; if basic compression pumps are prescribed (E0650; E0651), compression garments to protect abdomen/pelvis and chest should be worn during pumping.
  - Trial of complete decongestive therapy including manual lymphatic drainage
    - → referral to PT/certified lymphedema therapist
  - Monitor weight and anthropometrics (listed above) at every visit before any treatment to assess changes with therapy
- Referral to Pain Clinic and Wound Clinic, as needed
- SF-12 QoL Questionnaire at each MGH visit
- Consider plastic surgical consult if limited progress after 8–12 weeks of full compliance therapy

Graphic Summary

Stage	0	1	2	3
Diagnosis	Med. Evaluation, AFTD pitting test, venous duplex			
	Lymphoscintigraphy or ICG lymphography			
Treatment	Patient education and physical therapy			
	Weight loss and limb elevation			
	Compression garments (flat knit)			
	Compression pumps			Velcro*
	Benzopyrones			
	Manual lymphatic drainage			

Stage	0	1	2	3
Surgery		LVA		
			VLNT	
			SALP	
				Buried flap

Summary

Lymphedema management involves a comprehensive approach to reducing swelling and improving patients' quality of life. A multidisciplinary team is involved in all aspects of care. The protocol typically includes Complete Decongestive Therapy (CDT), which is divided into two phases: intensive and maintenance. The vascular team manages phlebolymphedema, while plastic and reconstructive surgery manage aspects of advanced stages of the disease. Our protocol includes initial workup, treatment, and monitoring.

Wounds: Protocol of Care 15

Maureen Walsh McCarthy
and Jeremy Goverman

Lower Extremity Venous Ulcer Treatment Algorithm

Full H&P

1. Diagnose wound(s): DDX mixed disease, PG, calciphylaxis, vasculitis, malignancy, etc.
   - Photo of wound(s), measurements
   - Assess pulses, edema, skin color/temp
   - Sx infection: NERDS (non-healing, exudate, red/friable, debris, smell = treat topically)
   - STONES (size, temp, os/bone, new breakdown, exudate/erythema/edema, smell = treat systemically)
   - Data: labs (including nutritional, inflammatory, A1C), imaging

M. W. McCarthy
Department of Surgery, Massachusetts General Hospital, Lead NP Wound Service, Boston, MA, USA
e-mail: Mmccarthy29@mgb.org

J. Goverman (✉)
Department of Surgery, Massachusetts General Hospital, Sumner Redstone Burn Center, Harvard Medical School, Boston, MA, USA
e-mail: jgoverman@mgh.harvard.edu

C. Echevarria et al. (eds.), *The Massachusetts General Hospital Protocols and Procedures for Venous Disease*,
https://doi.org/10.1007/978-3-032-05708-2_15

- Identify/address risk factors: immobility, hx trauma, DVT, congenital venous abnormality, CHF, age
- Note characteristic presentation: hemosiderin staining, lipodermatosclerosis, varicosities, dermatitis, location

Plan per Primary Team
- Antibiotics
- Management of comorbid conditions (DM, renal, resp, HF, etc.)
- Pain management

Orders
- XR, MRI r/o osteo
- Inflammatory markers
- nutrition labs (albumin, prealbumin, transferrin, H/H, …)
- Arterial LENIs * Vascular surgery consult as indicated

Wound Service Plan
- OR vs. bedside debridement: Urgent OR in case of extensive wounds, immunocompromised, or systemic symptoms (fever, leukocytosis, AMS, hypotension, tachycardia)
- Treat any associated cellulitis
- Topical wound care and treat dermatitis if present
- Consider NPWT and STSG
- Debride chronic wounds to reduce biofilm (chronic, no progress 2 weeks)
- Initiate compression, titrate up. Use bedside pneumatic pumps
- Cultures, consider obtaining biopsy
- Identify and control causative/contributing factors: DVT, tobacco use, obesity, sedentary
- Vascular surgery outpatient referral, venous duplex studies

References

CEAP classification (*C*linical signs, *E*tiology of venous disease, *A*natomic distribution, *P*athologic condition)

1. Reticular and spider veins
2. Varicose veins
3. Varicose veins and swelling

4. Varicose veins and evidence of venous stasis skin changes
5. Varicose veins and healed venous stasis ulceration
6. Varicose veins and an open venous ulceration

Lower Extremity Arterial Ulcer Treatment Algorithm

Full H&P

1. Diagnose wound(s): DDX mixed, pressure, calciphylaxis
   - Photo of wound(s), measurements
   - Assess pulses, edema, skin color/temp
   - Sx infection: NERDS (non-healing, exudate, red/friable, debris, smell=treat topically)
     STONES (size, temp, os/bone, new breakdown, exudate/erythema/edema, smell=treat systemically)
   - Data: labs (including nutritional, inflammatory, A1C), imaging
   - Identify/address risk factors: diabetes, PAD, smoking, age, HTN

Plan per Primary Team

- Antibiotics
- Management of comorbid conditions (DM, renal, resp, HF, etc.)
- Pain management

Orders

- XR, MRI r/o osteo
- Inflammatory markers
- A1C
- Nutrition labs (albumin, prealbumin, transferrin, H/H, …)
- Arterial LENIs * Vascular surgery consult
- Vascular surgery outpatient referral as indicated

Wound Service Plan

- OR vs. bedside debridement in setting of infection: Urgent OR in case of extensive wounds, immunocompromised, or systemic symptoms (fever, leukocytosis, AMS, hypotension, tachycardia)
- Topical wound care
- Leave dry stable eschar
- Debride chronic wounds to reduce biofilm (chronic, no progress 2 weeks)
- Cultures, ? biopsy
- Offloading, referral to brace shop

Neuropathic Foot Ulcer Treatment Algorithm

Full H&P

- Photo of wound(s)
- Correct grading, Wagner (Table 15.1), The University of Texas Staging System for Diabetic Foot Ulcers (Table 15.2)
- Monofilament testing: motor/sensory neuropathy
- Sx infection: NERDS (non-healing, exudate, red/friable, debris, smell=treat topically)
  STONES (size, temp, os/bone, new breakdown, exudate/erythema/edema, smell=treat systemically)

Table 15.1 Wagner classification

Grade.	Definition
Zero	No ulcer
One	Superficial skin ulcer
Two	Deep ulcer extending through dermis; tendon, ligaments, joint capsule, or bone may be exposed
Three	Deep ulcer with abscess, osteomyelitis or joint sepsis
Four	Localized gangrene (forefoot or heel)
Five	Gangrene of the foot

Table 15.2 The University of Texas staging system for diabetic foot ulcers

	Grade 0	Grade 1	Grade 2	Grade 3
Stage 1	Preulcerative or postulcerative lesions completely epithelialized	Superficial wound not involving tendon, capsule or bone	Wound penetrating tendon or capsule	Wound penetrating to bone or joint
Stage 2	Infection	Infection	Infection	Infection
Stage 3	Ischaemia	Ischaemia	Ischaemia	Ischaemia
Stage 4	Infection and Ischaemia	Infection and Ischaemia	Infection and Ischaemia	Infection and Ischaemia

- Data: labs (including nutritional, inflammatory, A1C), imaging
- Identify/address risk factors: mobility, edema, O_2 perfusion, PAD, glycemic control

Plan per Primary Team

- ID consult
- Antibiotics
- Management of comorbid conditions (DM, renal, resp, HF, smoking, etc.)

Orders

- XR, MRI r/o osteo
- Inflammatory markers
- Nutrition labs (albumin, prealbumin, transferrin, chol, H/H, Cr, etc.)
- A1C
- Arterial LENIs * Vascular surgery consult as indicated for revascularization
- Nutrition consult/ Endocrine/ Diab education
- Offloading, brace shop orders
- PT: mobility, esp. w new offloading Darco
- Activity, wt bear status, cane/crutches/walker/knee scooter/ wheelchair

Wound Service Plan

- OR vs. bedside debridement: Urgent OR in case of extensive wounds, immunocompromised, or systemic symptoms (fever, leukocytosis, AMS, hypotension, tachycardia)
- Topical wound care
- Debride chronic wounds to reduce biofilm (chronic, no progress 2 weeks)
- Cultures, biopsy

Discharge Plan

Wound clinic follow-up appointment

Referral to podiatry for definitive offloading (TCC, …) and prevention, surgical podiatry for corrective surgery

MGH Pressure Ulcer Treatment Plan

Full H&P

- Photo of wound(s)
- Correct staging
- Sx infection: NERDS (non-healing, exudate, red/friable, debris, smell = treat topically)
  STONES (size, temp, os/bone, new breakdown, exudate/erythema/edema, smell = treat systemically)
- Data: labs (including nutritional, inflammatory, A1C), imaging
- Identify/address risk factors: mobility, edema, O2 perfusion, incontinence, glycemic control

Plan per Primary Team

- ID consult
- Pain management
- Antibiotics
- Nutritional support (nocturnal feeds, NGT, GT)
- Management of comorbid conditions (DM, renal, resp, HF, etc.)

Orders

- XR, MRI r/o osteo
- Inflammatory markers
- nutrition labs (albumin, prealbumin, transferrin, chol, Cr …)
- Arterial LENIs if lower extremities
- Nutrition consult
- Support surface, offloading, frequent position changes
- PT: mobility, seating
- Activity, wt bear status

Wound Service Plan

- OR vs. bedside debridement: Urgent OR in case of extensive wounds, immunocompromised, or systemic symptoms (fever, leukocytosis, AMS, hypotension, tachycardia)
- Topical wound care
- Debride chronic wounds to reduce biofilm (chronic, no progress 2 weeks
- Cultures, biopsy
- ? Selection of objective criteria/tool for healing

Discharge Plan: Wound clinic follow-up appointment

Referral to spaulding wheelchair clinic for pressure mapping
Prevention (support surface at home …)

Summary

The *Wound Protocols chapter includes* lower extremity treatment algorithms that provide structured approaches for managing *venous, arterial, neuropathic, and pressure ulcers*, emphasizing *comprehensive assessment* and *multidisciplinary care*.

- *Venous Ulcers*: Focus on compression therapy, infection control (NERDS/STONES criteria), and addressing comorbidities (e.g., DVT, obesity).
- *Arterial Ulcers*: Prioritize *vascular evaluation* (pulses, imaging), offloading, and revascularization if needed.

- *Neuropathic Ulcers*: Use *Wagner/UT classifications*, glycemic control, offloading, and infection management.
- *Pressure Ulcers*: Stage wounds, optimize nutrition, and use *support surfaces* with frequent repositioning.

All protocols include information about:

- *Diagnostics*: Labs (A1C, inflammatory markers), imaging (XR/MRI), and wound cultures.
- *Interventions*: Debridement (bedside/OR), topical care, NPWT, and specialist referrals (vascular, podiatry).
- *Discharge Planning*: Wound clinic follow-up, patient education, and preventive measures.

Suggested Reading

Armstrong DG, American Diabetes Association, Lavery LA. Clinical care of the diabetic foot. 3rd ed. Alexandria: American Diabetes Association; 2016. Retrieved from https://phstwlp2.partners.org:3700/login.aspx?direct=true&db=nlebk&AN=1158394&site=eds-live&scope=site.

Aviles F. Charting a path to learning through an algorithm. Today's Wound Clinic. 2019;13(4) Retrieved from https://www.todayswoundclinic.com/articles/charting-path-learning-through-algorithm.

Hess CT. Venous ulcer assessment and management: using the updated CEAP classification system. Adv Skin Wound Care. 2020;33(11):614–5. https://doi.org/10.1097/01.ASW.0000719052.33284.73.

Kelechi TJ, Brunette G, Bonham PA, Crestodina L, Droste LR, Ratliff CR, Varnado MF. Guideline for management of wounds in patients with lower-extremity venous disease (LEVD). An executive summary. J Wound Ostomy Cont Nurs. 2019;47(2):97–110. https://doi.org/10.1097/WON.0000000000000622.

Kruger EA, Pires M, Ngann Y, Sterling M, Rubayi S. Comprehensive management of pressure ulcers in spinal cord injury: current concepts and future trends. J Spinal Cord Med. 2013;36(6):572–85. https://doi.org/10.1179/2045772313Y.0000000093.

National Pressure Ulcer Advisory Panel, European Pressure Ulcer Advisory Panel and Pan Pacific Pressure Injury Alliance. In: Haesler E, editor. Prevention and treatment of pressure ulcers: clinical practice guideline. Osborne Park: Cambridge Media; 2014. Retrieved from http://internationalguideline.com/static/pdfs/NPUAP-EPUAP-PPPIA-CPG-2017.pdf.

Snyder RJ, Jensen J, Applewhite AJ, Couch K, Joseph WS, Lantis Ii JC, Serena TE. A standardized approach to evaluating lower extremity chronic wounds using a checklist. Wounds. 2019;31(5 Suppl):S29–44. Retrieved from https://phstwlp2.partners.org:3700/login.aspx?direct=true&db=mdc&AN=31033453&site=eds-live&scope=site.

Weir GR, et al. Arterial disease ulcers, part 1: clinical diagnosis and investigation. Adv Skin Wound Care. 2014;27(9):421–8. https://doi.org/10.1097/01.ASW.0000453095.19109.5c.

Wound, Ostomy and Continence Nurses Society. 2019. Venous, arterial, and neuropathic lower-extremity wounds: clinical resource guide.

Part VI

Procedures

16 Vein Care Workflow: New Patient/Follow-Up

Carlos Echevarria, Sherry D. Scovell, and Julianne Stoughton

1. Retrieve patient from waiting area and bring to exam room
2. Verify patient's name and DOB
3. Have patient change into shorts
4. Take vitals
5. Take photos:
   (a) Anterior legs
   (b) Right leg toes out to the side
   (c) Left leg toes out to the side, left lateral leg
   (d) Right lateral leg
   (e) Posterior leg

C. Echevarria
Division of Vascular and Endovascular Surgery, Department of Surgery, Massachusetts General Hospital/Harvard Venous & Lymphatic Medicine Alumni, Boston, MA, USA

Division of Vascular Medicine and Endovenous Interventions, Veins & Vascular Centers of Excellence, Phoenix, AZ, USA
e-mail: carlos.echevarria@vascular.md

S. D. Scovell · J. Stoughton (✉)
Division of Vascular and Endovascular Surgery, Department of Surgery, Massachusetts General Hospital/Harvard Medical School, Boston, MA, USA
e-mail: sscovell@mgh.harvard.edu; jstoughton@mgh.harvard.edu

C. Echevarria et al. (eds.), *The Massachusetts General Hospital Protocols and Procedures for Venous Disease*,
https://doi.org/10.1007/978-3-032-05708-2_16

6. Enter the patient's chart in EHR
7. *Rooming*—complete the following sections:
   (a) Reason for visit (varicose veins, pain, follow-up)
   (b) Enter vitals
   (c) Enter OB/GYN status (mark as reviewed)
   (d) Reconcile medications (mark as reviewed)
   (e) Reconcile allergies (mark as reviewed)
   (f) Enter medical history/conditions (include all history, not just vascular)
   (g) Vascular history
   (h) Medical history (mark as reviewed)
   (i) Surgical history (mark as reviewed)
   (j) Family history—check off any family member with pertinent conditions (mark as reviewed)
   (k) Smoking/alcohol intake (mark as reviewed)
8. *Obstetric history:*
   (a) Chart review
   (b) Medical history
   (c) Obstetrics
   (d) Enter gravida (how many pregnancies)
   (e) Enter para (how many live births)
   (f) Record outcome data for each (mark as reviewed)
9. *Plan:*
   (a) Enter visit diagnosis
   (b) Enter a new order for compression stockings, if needed, under Medications and Orders
   (c) Talk to patient about compression stockings/measure if needed
10. *Note*
   (a) +create note
   (b) Populate all of the rooming tab into note
   (c) Fill out blank symptoms
   (d) Compression stockings—fill out accordingly
   (e) Medical history
   (f) Social history—job/standing/sitting/exercise
   (g) GYN history—hormone replacement therapy
   (h) Review of systems
   (i) VCSS

   (j) CEAP—enter according to chart
   (k) Close note—sign on close encounter
11. *Wrap Up*
   (a) Patient instructions—enter instructions for upcoming treatment/follow-up
   (b) Provide patient with compression hose vendor/online list
12. After visit is complete with physician take patient to the appropriate scheduling area (front desk or surgery scheduler)

Vein Care Workflow for Procedures: Radiofrequency Ablation, EVLT, Varithena, MOCA

1. Retrieve the patient from the waiting area and escort to procedure room
2. Verify patient's name and DOB/confirm consents are signed and universal protocol is filled out
3. Have patient change into gown, underwear (men two pair), and socks
4. Take photos:
   (a) Anterior legs
   (b) Right leg toes out to side
   (c) Left leg toes out to the side
   (d) Left lateral leg
   (e) Right lateral leg
   (f) Posterior leg
5. Complete white board
6. Enter the patient's details in EHR
7. *Rooming:*
   (a) Reason for visit
   (b) Take and enter vitals
   (c) Reconcile medications (mark as reviewed)
   (d) Reconcile allergies (mark as reviewed)
   (e) Verify medical history/enter medical condition (mark as reviewed)
   (f) Enter the surgery for today in chart review (with the date, leg, and vein) (mark as reviewed)

(g) Enter family history (mark as reviewed)
(h) Smoking history (mark as reviewed)
(i) Alcohol intake (mark as reviewed)
(j) Change status to green notifying the physician patient is ready

8. *Plan:*
   (a) Enter diagnosis
   (b) Enter a new order for compression stockings under Medications and Orders if needed
9. *Note tab:*
   (a) +create note
   (b) Procedure
   (c) Physician
   (d) Assistant
   (e) Anesthesia (include ml used of tumescent)
   (f) Medications taken for procedure
   (g) VCSS/CEAP
   (h) Duraprep/Chloraprep
   (i) Record appropriate information according to procedure

   RF—vein, time, centimeters, cycles in table provided

   EVLT—name of vein treatment time in seconds, Joules, length of treated segment

   Varithena—amount purged, amount drawn, amount administered in total

   (j) Incisions and sites
   (k) Procedure start and end time
   (l) Whom patient was released to
   (m) Compression hose used
   (n) Sign on close encounter
10. *Radiofrequency* (RF) steps for procedure:
   (a) Place generator in the procedure room
   (b) Retrieve catheter from supply area according to physician initials marked on the box
   (c) Place ultrasound in room—enter first and last name with MRN
   (d) Large surgical pack—add all supplies according to set-up sheet

(e) Fill bags with tumescent (according to set-up instructions), place bag on top of pump
(f) Sheath (micro introducer sheath)
(g) Place the catheter sticker, MIS lot number, and expiration on the bottom of the protocol timeout sheet
(h) Have a vein light and marking pen on hand if ambulatory phlebectomy (AP) involved
(i) Make sure "hardstop" is completed
(j) Assist physician prepping patient if needed
(k) Obtain ice in sterile bag for procedure
(l) Connect the catheter to the generator
(m) Talk with the patient during the procedure
(n) Assist in the procedure
(o) Assist physician with dressings if needed
(p) Assist patient with compression stockings
(q) Offer the patient a snack/drink
(r) Re-take vitals
(s) Record information from generator into note
(t) Finish note—sign on close encounter
(u) At appropriate time patient may proceed to get dressed
(v) Clean the procedure room

11. *Endovenous Laser Treatment (EVLT)* steps for procedure:
(a) Place laser in the procedure room
(b) Retrieve laser fiber from the supply area
(c) Have goggles accessible
(d) Hang "caution: laser in use" sign on outside of door
(e) Place ultrasound in room—enter first and last name with MRN
(f) Large surgical pack—add all supplies according to set-up sheet
(g) Fill bags with tumescent (according to set-up instructions), place bag on top of pump
(h) 4F micropuncture kit
(i) Place the laser sticker, 4F micropuncture lot number, and expiration date at the bottom of the protocol timeout sheet
(j) Have a vein light and a vein marking pen on hand if AP involved

(k) Make sure "hardstop" is completed
(l) Assist physician prepping patient if needed
(m) Obtain ice for procedure
(n) Assist in the procedure
(o) Talk with the patient during the procedure
(p) Assist physician with dressings if needed
(q) Assist patient with compression stockings
(r) Offer the patient a snack and drink
(s) Re-take vitals
(t) Record information from laser into note
(u) Finish note—sign on close encounter
(v) At appropriate time patient may proceed to get dressed
(w) Clean the procedure room

12. *Ambulatory Phlebectomy (AP)* steps for procedure:
    (a) Small surgical pack—add all supplies according to set-up sheet
    (b) Fill bags with tumescent (according to set-up instructions), place bag on top of pump
    (c) Have a vein light and a marking pen on hand
    (d) Make sure "hardstop" is completed
    (e) Assist physician prepping patient if needed
    (f) Talk to the patient during the procedure
    (g) Assist physician with dressings if needed
    (h) Assist physician with Steri-Strips/Tegaderm/ABD pads over incisions
    (i) Assist patient with compression stocking
    (j) Offer the patient a snack/drink
    (k) Re-take vitals
    (l) Record areas of incisions into the note
    (m) Finish note—sign on close encounter
    (n) At the appropriate time patient may proceed to get dressed
    (o) Clean the procedure room
13. *Polidocanol endovenous microfoam (Varithena)* steps for procedure:
    (a) Two medical assistants must be present—1 sterile and 1 circulator

(b) Large surgical pack—add all supplies according to set-up sheet
(c) Obtain the canister and administrator pack, place on the counter in procedure room
(d) Flush dilator, sheath, and tubing
(e) Make sure "hardstop" is completed
(f) Assist physician prepping patient if needed
(g) Talk to the patient during the procedure
(h) Assist physician with procedure
(i) Circulator holds canister and enters information onto the log during procedure
(j) Record veins injected, amount of purged, amount used and indications (follow same protocol for US-guided sclerotherapy and indicate veins injected, solution, form, and amount where ultrasound was used)
(k) Follow instruction from the physician for how long patient should stay laying down
(l) Assist patient with compression stockings and bolsters
(m) Offer the patient a snack/drink
(n) Re-take vitals
(o) Record information from log into the note
(p) Finish note—sign on close encounter
(q) At the appropriate time patient may proceed to get dressed
(r) Clean the procedure room

14. *MOCA (ClariVein)* steps for procedure:
(a) Place ClariVein kit in the procedure room
(b) Place ultrasound in room—enter first and last name with MRN
(c) Large surgical pack—add all supplies according to set-up sheet
(d) Add prepared 1% and 3% STS
(e) Place the ClariVein sticker, 4F micropuncture lot number, and expiration on the bottom of the protocol timeout sheet
(f) Have a vein light and marking pen on hand if AP involved
(g) Make sure "hardstop" is completed
(h) Assist physician prepping patient if needed

(i) Talk with the patient during the procedure
(j) Assist physician with dressings if needed
(k) Assist patient with compression stockings
(l) Offer the patient a snack/drink
(m) Re-take vitals
(n) Record information from procedure into the note
(o) Finish note—sign on close encounter
(p) At appropriate time patient may proceed to get dressed
(q) Clean the procedure room

15. *Wrap up tab:*
    (a) Patient is given post-procedure instructions (AVS)

Rooming a Post-Op

- Bring patient to the room
- Have patient change into shorts
- Take vitals
- Start by entering patient's chart
- Rooming:
  1. Reason for visit (varicose veins, pain, and post-op)
  2. Enter vitals
  3. Reconcile meds
  4. Reconcile allergies
  5. Enter medical history/enter medical conditions
  6. Enter venous info related to DVT/ EDEMA/ PAIN/ PHLEBITIS/ULCER/VARICOSE VEINS/VENOUS SUFFICIENCY
  7. Enter past surgical history
  8. Enter family history—varicose veins and Clotting Disorder
  9. Smoking history
  10. Alcohol intake
- Plan Tab:
  1. Enter diagnosis (varicose veins with pain, varicose veins with edema, venous insufficiency)
- Note:
  1. + Create post-procedure progress note
  2. Enter post op days

3. Enter procedure
4. Enter complaints
5. Enter physical exam
6. Enter venous ultrasound if needed
7. Sign on close encounter

- Wrap up:
  1. Enter instructions if needed
  2. Enter level of Service
  3. Enter physician who did the procedure
  4. Sign on close encounter

Summary

The *Vein Care Workflow* outlines standardized procedures for new/follow-up patients and vein treatments (e.g., radiofrequency ablation, EVLT, Varithena, MOCA). For *new patients*, steps include intake (vitals, photos, EHR documentation), comprehensive history-taking (medical, vascular, obstetric), and care planning (compression stockings, follow-ups). *Procedures* follow strict protocols: patient prep, consent verification, imaging, EHR documentation, and post-op instructions. Each treatment has specific setup requirements (equipment, tumescent solution, safety checks) and intra-procedure tasks (assisting physicians, recording data). Post-op visits include recovery tracking, vitals, and ultrasound checks if needed.

Thermal Ablation Techniques

17

Carlos Echevarria, Sherry D. Scovell, and Julianne Stoughton

Endovenous Ablation Set Up

Set Up

Ultrasound on and patient name in
Veinlite and pen
1 large surgical pack
1 pair of sterile gloves
1 stick of DuraPrep/ChloraPrep
1 package of tubing
1 25″ gauge needle

C. Echevarria
Division of Vascular and Endovascular Surgery, Department of Surgery, Massachusetts General Hospital/Harvard Venous & Lymphatic Medicine Alumni, Boston, MA, USA

Division of Vascular Medicine and Endovenous Interventions, Veins & Vascular Centers of Excellence, Phoenix, AZ, USA
e-mail: carlos.echevarria@vascular.md

S. D. Scovell · J. Stoughton (✉)
Division of Vascular and Endovascular Surgery, Department of Surgery, Massachusetts General Hospital/Harvard Medical School, Boston, MA, USA
e-mail: sscovell@mgh.harvard.edu; jstoughton@mgh.harvard.edu

C. Echevarria et al. (eds.), *The Massachusetts General Hospital Protocols and Procedures for Venous Disease*,
https://doi.org/10.1007/978-3-032-05708-2_17

250 mL saline bag
1 ice bag
1 elastic
1 Tegaderm
2 stopcocks (PEM)
1 extra tubing 4 in (PEM)
If phlebectomy add:
2 jakes baby hemostat
1 scissors
1 light cover
1 micro needle
Steri-Strips
All procedures need:
1 fluid bag ready to mix tumescent (includes sodium bicarb and 1% lidocane with epi)
1 gown
1 pair of socks
1 underwear (men get 2 pairs)
1 large ACE wrap
1 goodie bag (small ACE bandage, ABD pad, ice pack, instructions)

Open the large kit first and sterilely place all components on the table at least 5 inches above the sterile field, carefully not contaminating any of the supplies. It does not matter which order they are placed on the table. During this procedure you will have to obtain ice from the machine or freezer (ice in a sterile bag is used for vasoconstriction and pain control). Talk to the patient, keep them calm and relaxed. Make sure there is music the patient prefers and, if not, something soothing (classical is a good go-to).

Make sure the patient is appropriately dressed for the procedure; there is a Veinlite and marking pen for marking. Ask the patient about meds, allergies, and DOB every time. Sedatives are optional, but recommended in thermal procedures. Patients cannot drive if they took sedatives. Identify the designated driver prior to initiating the procedure. Compression hoses are needed for every procedure.

Radiofrequency Ablation Note

@NAME@
@MRN@
@ED@

PRE-PROCEDURE DIAGNOSIS:
{Blank single:19197::"Right","Left","Bilateral"} leg venous insufficiency with varicose veins, leg pain, and edema

POST-PROCEDURE DIAGNOSIS: Same

PROCEDURE:
{Blank single:19197::"Right","Left","Bilateral"} leg Radiofrequency Catheter ablation of the {Blank multiple:19196::"great saphenous","anterior accessory saphenous","small saphenous","posterior thigh extension"} vein.
{Blank single:19197::"Right","Left","Bilateral"} leg ambulatory phlebectomy *** microincisions

PHYSICIAN: Carlos Echevarria, MD

FELLOW: ***

ASSISTANT: {Blank single:19197::"xyz","xyz"}

Surgical History:
@PSH@

ANESTHESIA:
1% lidocaine
*** mL Tumescent local ({Blank multiple:19196::"250 mL .09% sodium chloride, 10 cc lidocaine with epinephrine, and 2.5 cc sodium bicarbonate","500 mL .09% sodium chloride, 20 cc lidocaine with epinephrine, and 5 cc sodium bicarbonate"})

Medications:
@MEDENC@
{Blank multiple:19196::"Cefadroxil 500 mg","Cefadroxil 1000 mg","Clindamycin 600 mg","Valium 5 mg", "Valium 10 mg","Lorazepam 0.5 mg","Lorazepam 1 mg","Lovenox 30 mg", "Lovenox 40 mg":}

Allergies:
@ALG@

VITAL SIGNS:
@VITALSMULTIPLE@

@TIMEOUT@

PROCEDURE START TIME: ***

VCSS: R:*** L:***
CEAP CLASS: Right: {Blank single:19197::"C0","C1","C2","C 3","C4","C5","C6"} Left:{Blank single:19197::"C0","C1","C 2","C3","C4","C5","C6"}

INDICATIONS: @DIAG@
Leg pain, swelling, varicose veins, and venous insufficiency in the {Blank single:19197::"right","left","bilateral"} leg {Blank multiple:19196::"great saphenous","anterior accessory saphenous","small saphenous","posterior thigh extension"} vein system. Conservative measures failed (hose, elevation, exercise, medications).

FINDINGS:
The treated saphenous vein(s) appeared to be occluded following the ablation procedure, although the view was limited secondary to tumescent anesthesia. The common femoral and popliteal veins were normal and compressible after the procedure. There were no phlebitic vein segments. The *** vein is enlarged and refluxing from the *** to the *** level.

PROCEDURE:

The patient was placed in the {Blank multiple:19196::"supine","prone","left lateral decubitus","right lateral decubitus"} position on the operating table; the {Blank single:19197::"right","left","bilateral"} leg was prepped with {Blank single:19197:: "DuraPrep", "ChloraPrep"} and draped sterilely. An intraoperative ultrasound was performed with the above findings. A small injection of 1% Xylocaine was made in the skin, and a 21-gauge thin-walled needle was used to insert into the {Blank multiple:19196::"great saphenous","anterior accessory saphenous","small saphenous","posterior thigh extension"} vein at the *** level, using ultrasound guidance, and a 0.018 glide wire was inserted and advanced toward the saphenous junction using ultrasound guidance.

The 7 French dilator and sheath were advanced over the wire after being irrigated with saline. The 7 French radio frequency catheter was advanced over the wire, infused with saline, and the tip of the catheter was properly positioned just beyond the first-order branch of the {Blank multiple:19196::"great saphenous","anterior accessory saphenous","small saphenous","posterior thigh extension"} vein using ultrasound guidance. The patient was placed in Trendelenburg position. Tumescent anesthesia was administered along the length of the catheter using ultrasound guidance; the generator was used to treat the vein along its length, applying pressure as it was withdrawn. {Blank multiplc:19196::"3.0", "6.5"} cm segments were treated (proximal to distal) for 20 s each using the following:

vein treated	proximal to distal	total cycles	total length	total time
***	***	***	***	***

vein treated	proximal to distal	total cycles	total length	total time
***	***	***	***	***

The post-procedure ultrasound was done with the above findings. The catheter and sheath were withdrawn, and pressure was held for hemostasis.

The previously marked varicose veins of the {Blank single:19 197::"right","left","bilateral"} leg were infused with tumescent anesthesia. A total of *** micro-incisions were made to remove the symptomatic varicosities in the following areas ***. All the incisions were dressed with Steri-Strips and Tegaderm. ABD pads were placed over each incision site, and a 30 mmHg compression stocking ({Blank multiple:19196::"thigh high", "thigh high with waist attachment","Pantyhose","knee high"}) was applied on the patient. An additional ACE bandage was applied over the stockings to the high-thigh level, to be taken off prior to bedtime.

PROCEDURE END TIME:***

DISCHARGE:

Estimated blood loss was minimal, all counts were correct, and the patient's prognosis for recovery is good. There were no complications. There were no specimens sent. The patient will leave their compression stocking on until the post-procedure visit and then for the remainder of 2 weeks during waking hours, or as directed by the physician. The patient ambulated upon discharge after having tolerated the procedure well. Oral and written instructions were reviewed with the patient before discharge. The patient was released to *** and will plan to return in 1–2 days for an ultrasound and dressing change.

Perforator Ablation Set-Up

Set Up

Ultrasound on and patient name in
Sterile pen
1 large surgical pack
1 pair of sterile gloves
1 stick of DurapPrep/ChloraPrep
1 lidocaine 1%
1 25″ gauge needle

1 18″ gauge peripheral IV catheter
250 mL saline bag
1 ice bag
1 elastic
1 Steri-Strips
All procedures need:
1 Fluid bag ready to mix tumescent (includes sodium bicarb and 1% lidocane with epi)
1 gown
1 pair of socks
1 underwear (men get 2 pairs)
1 large ACE wrap
1 goodie bag (small ACE bandage, ABD pad, ice pack, instructions)

Open the large kit first and sterilely place all components on the table at least 5 inches above the sterile field, carefully not contaminating any of the supplies. It does not matter which order they are placed on the table. During this procedure you will have to obtain ice from a machine or freezer (ice in a sterile bag is used for vasoconstriction and pain control). Talk to the patient, keep them calm and relaxed. Make sure there is music the patient prefers and, if not, something soothing (classical is a good go-to).

Make sure the patient is appropriately dressed for the procedure. Ask patients meds, allergies, DOB, every time. Sedatives are optional but recommended in thermal procedures. Patients cannot drive if they took sedatives. Identify the designated driver prior to initiating the procedure. Compression hoses are needed for every procedure.

Endovenous Laser Ablation of Pathological Perforator Note

NOTE NAME-
DOB-

MRN-

PRE-PROCEDURE DIAGNOSIS: {::"right","left","bilateral"} leg venous insufficiency with varicose veins, leg pain and edema

POST-PROCEDURE DIAGNOSIS: Same PROCEDURE: {::"right","left","bilateral"} leg endovenous laser ablation of the perforator vein ___ cm from malleolus.

PHYSICIAN: Carlos Echevarria, MD

ASSISTANT:

ANESTHESIA: 1% lidocaine ____ mL Tumescent local

500mL 0.9% sodium chloride, 20cc lidocaine 1% and 5cc sodium bicarbonate

1000ml 0.9% sodium chloride, 40 cc lidocaine 1%, and 10 cc sodium bicarbonate

500 mL 0.9% sodium chloride, 10 cc lidocaine 2%, and 5 cc sodium bicarbonate

PERI-OPMEDICATIONS:??{Blankmultiple:19196::"Cefadroxil 500mg","Cefadroxil 1000mg","Clindamycin 600mg","Valium 5mg", "Valium 10 mg","Lorazepam 0.5mg","Lorazepam 1mg","Lovenox 30mg", "Lovenox 40mg":}

ALLERGIES: VITAL SIGNS: BP ___ HR ___

-TIMEOUT-

PROCEDURE START TIME: ___

INDICATIONS:Leg pain, swelling, varicose veins, and venous insufficiency in the {::"right","left","bilateral"} leg perforator vein. Conservative measures failed (hose, elevation, exercise, medications).

FINDINGS: The treated perforator vein appeared to be occluded following the ablation procedure, although the view was limited secondary to tumescent anesthesia. The deep venous system is normal and compressible after the procedure. There were no phlebitic vein segments. The vein in question is enlarged and refluxing from the DEEP VENOUS SYSTEM to the SUPERFICIAL level.

PROCEDURE:Thepatientwasplacedinthe{"supine","prone","left lateral decubitus","right lateral decubitus"} position on the operating table; the {Blank single:19197::"right","left","bilateral"} leg was prepped with {"isopropyl alcohol 70%", "duraprep", "chloraprep"} and draped sterilely. An intraoperative ultrasound was performed with the above findings. A small injection of lidocaine was made in the skin, and an 18-gauge peripheral IV catheter was used to insert into the PERFORATOR vein at the SUPERFICIAL level, using ultrasound guidance. The catheter was inserted and advanced within the perforator using ultrasound guidance. Using Seldinger technique, the laser fiber was placed and positioned properly within the perforator vein in question. 20 mL of tumescent solution was administered perivenously. The total length of the perforator vein was treated at the fascia level. The patient was placed in Trendelenburg position. Tumescent anesthesia was administered along the length of the catheter using ultrasound guidance.

vein treated: ___ perforator vein ___ cm from malleolus
total Energy: ___ Joules
total length: 1 cm
total time: 10 sec(s)
tumescent anesthesia used:___ mL

The post-procedure ultrasound was done with the above findings. The fiber and catheter were withdrawn, and pressure was held for hemostasis. Gauze pads were placed over each incision site and a 20–30 mmHg compression stocking ({:"thigh high", "thigh high with waist attachment","Pantyhose","knee high"}) was applied on the patient. An additional ace bandage was applied over stockings to the high thigh level to be taken off prior to bedtime. PROCEDURE END TIME: ___

POST-OP VITALS:

- DISCHARGE: Estimated blood loss is minimal, all counts were correct, and the patient's prognosis for recovery is good. There were no complications. There were no specimens sent. The patient will leave their compression stocking on until the post-procedure visit and then for the remainder of 2 weeks during waking hours or as directed by the physician. The patient ambulated upon discharge after having tolerated the procedure well. Oral and written instructions were reviewed with the patient before discharge. The patient expressed understanding of instructions given regarding compression stockings (i.e., improve the procedure success rate, ongoing use for 48 h, and during the day only for 2 weeks). The patient was released to ___ and will plan to return in 1–2 days for an ultrasound and dressing change.

Summary

The *Endovenous Ablation Setup and Documentation* outlines standardized protocols for *radiofrequency ablation (RFA)* and *endovenous laser ablation (EVLA)* of saphenous and perforator veins. Key steps include the following:

- *Pre-procedure setup*: Ultrasound initialization, sterile kit preparation, tumescent anesthesia, surgical prep, and patient verification (medications, allergies, consent).
- *Procedure details*: Catheter/fiber insertion under ultrasound guidance, tumescent administration, vein ablation (segment length, energy delivery), and post-procedure occlusion confirmation.
- *Post-op care*: Compression stockings, wound dressings (Steri-Strips, Tegaderm), and discharge instructions (activity, follow-up ultrasound).

Perforator ablation follows a similar workflow, with an emphasis on targeting refluxing pathological perforators. Documentation templates ensure consistency, capturing diagnoses, anesthesia, vitals, and procedural metrics (e.g., joules, tumescent volume).

Non-thermal Ablation Techniques

18

Carlos Echevarria, Sherry D. Scovell, and Julianne Stoughton

Polidocanol Microfoam (Varithena)

Set Up

Ultrasound on and patient name in
Veinlite and pen
1 Large surgical pack
Varithena Admin pack
Varithena cannister

C. Echevarria
Division of Vascular and Endovascular Surgery, Department of Surgery, Massachusetts General Hospital/Harvard Venous & Lymphatic Medicine Alumni, Boston, MA, USA

Division of Vascular Medicine and Endovenous Interventions, Veins & Vascular Centers of Excellence, Phoenix, AZ, USA
e-mail: carlos.echevarria@vascular.md

S. D. Scovell · J. Stoughton (✉)
Division of Vascular and Endovascular Surgery, Department of Surgery, Massachusetts General Hospital/Harvard Medical School, Boston, MA, USA
e-mail: sscovell@mgh.harvard.edu; jstoughton@mgh.harvard.edu

C. Echevarria et al. (eds.), *The Massachusetts General Hospital Protocols and Procedures for Venous Disease*,
https://doi.org/10.1007/978-3-032-05708-2_18

1 pair of sterile gloves
1 stick of DuraPrep/ChloraPrep
1 25″ gauge needle
1 ice bag
1 elastic
1 Tegaderm
1 scissors
1 light cover
Steri-Strips
2 stopcocks
1 extra tubing 4 in
250 ml saline bag
All procedures need:
1 gown
1 pair of socks
1 underwear (men get 2 pairs)
1 large ACE wrap
1 goodie bag (small ACE bandage, chux, ABD pad, ice pack, instructions)

Open the large surgical pack first and sterilely place all components on the table at least 5 inches above the sterile field, carefully not contaminating any of the supplies. It does not matter which order they are placed on the table. During this procedure you will have to obtain ice from machine or freezer (ice in a sterile bag is used for vasoconstriction and pain control). Talk to the patient to keep them calm and relaxed. Make sure there is music the patient prefers and, if not, something soothing (classical is a good go-to).

Make sure the patient is appropriately dressed for the procedure. Ask patients about meds, allergies, and DOB every time. Sedatives are optional. Patients cannot drive if they took sedatives. Identify the designated driver prior to initiating the procedure. Compression hoses are needed for every procedure.

Polidocanol Endovenous Microfoam (Varithena) Note

@NAME@
@MRN@
@ED@

PRE-PROCEDURE DIAGNOSIS:{Blank single:19197::"Right", "Left","Bilateral"} leg venous insufficiency with varicose veins, leg pain, and edema

POST-PROCEDURE DIAGNOSIS: Same

PROCEDURE:
{Blank single:19197::"Right","Left","Bilateral"} leg Varithena Foam of the following veins: {Blank multiple:19196::"great saphenous","anterior accessory saphenous","small saphenous","posterior thigh extension","tributaries"}

PHYSICIAN: Carlos Echevarria, MD

FELLOW: ***

ASSISTANT: {Blank multiple:19196::"xyz ","xyz"}

Surgical History:
@PSH@

ANESTHESIA:
Local 1% lidocaine cutaneous anesthetic

Medications:
@MEDENC@
{Blank multiple:19196::"Cefadroxil 500 mg","Cefadroxil 1000 mg","Clindamycin 600 mg","Valium 5 mg", "Valium 10 mg","Lorazepam 0.5 mg","Lorazepam 1 mg":}

Allergies:
@ALG@

VITALS:
@VITALSMULTIPLE@

POST-OP VITALS:
BP:*** Pulse:***

@TIMEOUT@

PROCEDURE START TIME: ***

VCSS: R:*** L:***
CEAP CLASS: Right: {Blank single:19197::"C0","C1","C2","C3","C4","C5","C6"} Left:{Blank single:19197::"C0","C1","C2","C3","C4","C5","C6"}

INDICATIONS:
@DIAG@
Leg pain, swelling, varicose veins, and venous insufficiency in the {Blank single:19197::"right","left","bilateral"} leg {Blank multiple:19196::"great saphenous","anterior accessory saphenous","posterior thigh extension"} vein system. Conservative measures failed (hose, elevation, exercise, medications). Polidocanol endovenous microfoam (Varithena®) is indicated for the treatment of incompetent great saphenous veins, accessory saphenous veins, and visible varicosities of the saphenous vein system above and below the knee. Varithena® improves the symptoms of superficial venous incompetence and the appearance of visible varicosities.

FINDINGS:
The treated saphenous vein(s) appeared to be occluded following the Varithena Foam procedure. The common femoral and popliteal veins were normal and compressible after the procedure. There were no phlebitic vein segments. The *** vein is enlarged and refluxing from the *** to the *** level.

PROCEDURE:

1. Microfoam chemical ablation with Varithena of the {Blank single:19197::"right","left","bilateral"} {Blank multiple:19196::"great saphenous","anterior accessory saphenous","small saphenous","posterior thigh extension"} from *** to the *** access site.
2. Intraoperative ultrasound guidance.

The patient walked to the procedure room. All applicable staff donned appropriate apparel. A procedure time out was performed to confirm correct patient, correct extremity, correct procedure, and correct room set, including presence of all applicable supplies, devices, and drugs. A duplex ultrasound scan confirmed the location and incompetence of the refluxing veins, and their course was marked on the skin together with the dilated tributaries. Incompetent perforating veins *** identified. The extent of treatment of the target veins and the associated varicosities was determined through US mapping by the treating physician.

The patient was placed on the OR table {Blank multiple:19196::"supine","prone","left lateral decubitus","right lateral decubitus"} and was evaluated in reverse Trendelenburg position. The limb was prepped with *** and sterile drapes were applied. A skin wheal was made to facilitate access using 1.0% lidocaine at the chosen puncture site. The skin was punctured through the anesthetized skin with the venous access needle and advanced under ultrasound guidance into the vein to be treated with a micropuncture needle, followed by passage of a 0.018 guide wire through the needle. For the truncal veins, a 4 French dilator sheath was placed over the wire and flushed with saline. Catheter access was established for each of the target vessels and venous access confirmed by aspiration of dark, low-pressure blood. Upon gaining all access sites, both above and below the knee, the target limb was positioned at 45 degrees of elevation in relationship to the torso.

The Varithena canister was activated, and the canister was primed and purged as required in the instructions for use. Aliquots of Varithena foam were drawn into a sterile syringe, which was then attached to a heparinized, saline-filled extension tube for administration of Varithena through the extension tube into the vascular catheter. Varithena was slowly administered at 0.5–1.0 cc/s with close observation by ultrasound of its course in the Veins. When the Varithena foam arrived to approximately 3–5 cm from the deep vein junction, the target vein was then compressed to prevent flow into the deep system. Further administration of Varithena was stopped at this point, and the treated veins were observed with ultrasound over a period of 3–5 min, observing for spasm, and cessation of proximal flow was established. The other veins were then treated in the same manner, repeating the steps above (see chart below). At this point, previously marked dilated varicosities were treated using image guidance and direct puncture until all varices had been successfully treated or when a maximum volume of Varithena had been reached. During administration of Varithena, the patient was asked to dorsiflex the ankle to limit flow of foam into perforating veins. Once appropriate spasm had been confirmed in the treated veins, the vascular catheter was removed from the leg, and light pressure was applied over the puncture site for hemostasis.

The common femoral and deep superficial veins were then evaluated for flow and compressibility prior to dressing placement. The lower extremity was kept elevated at 45 degrees above the horizontal, and cording material {Blank multiple:19196::"was","was not"} applied over the saphenous segments and tributaries to allow for eccentric compression over the target vessels, including the targeted saphenous vein(s).

The patient ambulated for 10 min under supervision and was without apparent concerns at the time of release. Post-care instructions include walking 5 min of every waking hour, wearing compression 24 h per day, taking it off only to shower and then reapplying for 2 weeks. The patient was instructed to take an anti-inflammatory medicine as needed and to follow up for a color duplex scan of the GSV, the treated superficial varices, the adjacent deep veins, and additional treatment as needed.

4F Sheath:

Vein treated	Entry site	Amount purged	Amount drawn	Amount administered
***	***	***	***	***

Vein treated	Entry site	Amount purged	Amount drawn	Amount administered
***	***	***	***	***

US Guidance

Direct Inject:

Vein treated	Amount purged	Amount drawn	Amount administered
***	***	***	***

Vein treated	Amount purged	Amount drawn	Amount administered
***	***	***	***

Vein treated	Amount purged	Amount drawn	Amount administered
***	***	***	***

The post-procedure ultrasound was performed with the above findings. The catheter and sheath were withdrawn, and pressure was held for hemostasis.

The leg was lowered only after compression had been applied and the patient was immediately ambulatory. All the incisions were dressed with steri-strips and tegaderm. ABD pads were placed over each incision site and a 30 mmHg compression stocking {Blank multiple:19196::"Thigh High","Thigh High with waist attachment","Pantyhose"} was applied on the patient. An additional ACE bandage was applied over stockings to the high thigh level to be taken off prior to bed time.

PROCEDURE END TIME: ***

DISCHARGE/PLAN:

Estimated blood loss is minimal, all counts were correct, and the patient's prognosis for recovery is good. There were no complications. There were no specimens sent. The patient will leave their compression stocking on until the post procedure visit and then for a remainder of 2 weeks during waking hours, or as directed by the physician. The patient ambulated upon discharge after having tolerated the procedure well. Oral and written instructions were reviewed with the patient before discharge. The patient was released to *** and will plan to return in 1–2 days for an ultrasound and dressing change. The patient will be scheduled for further injections of varithena as needed for residual varices or truncal reflux in the next 4–6 weeks as needed.

Cyanocrylate Glue (VenaSeal)/Mechanochemical Ablation (MOCA)

Set Up

Ultrasound on and patient name in
Veinlite and pen
1 Large surgical pack
VenaSeal-Glue kit
1 pair of sterile gloves
1 stick of DuraPrep/ChlorPprep
1 25″ gauge needle
1 ice bag
1 elastic
1 Tegaderm
1 scissors
Steri-Strips
2 stopcocks

250 ml saline bag
All procedures need:
1 gown
1 pair of socks
1 underwear (men get 2 pairs)
1 large ACE wrap
1 goodie bag (small ACE bandage, chux, ABD pad, ice pack, instructions)

Open the large kit first and sterilely place all components on the table at least 5 inches above the sterile field, carefully not contaminating any of the supplies. It does not matter which order they are placed on the table. During this procedure you will have to obtain ice from the machine or freezer (ice in a sterile bag is used for vasoconstriction and pain control). Talk to the patient; keep them calm and relaxed. Make sure there is music the patient prefers and, if not, something soothing (classical is a good go-to).

Make sure the patient is appropriately dressed for the procedure; there is a Veinlite and marking pen for marking. Ask patients about meds, allergies, and DOB every time. Sedatives are optional. Patients cannot drive if they took sedatives. Identify the designated driver prior to initiating the procedure. Compression hoses are needed for every procedure.

Cyanoacrylate Glue (VenaSeal) Note

@NAME@
@MRN@
@ED@

PRE-PROCEDURE DIAGNOSIS:{Blank single:19197::"Right", "Left","Bilateral"} leg venous insufficiency with varicose veins, leg pain, and edema

POST-PROCEDURE DIAGNOSIS: Same

PROCEDURE:
{Blank single:19197::"Right","Left","Bilateral"} leg VenaSeal Glue of the following veins: {Blank multiple:19196::"great saphenous","anterior great saphenous","small saphenous","posterior thigh extension","tributaries"}

PHYSICIAN: Carlos Echevarria, MD

FELLOW: ***

ASSISTANT: {Blank multiple:19196::"xyz ","xyz"}

Surgical History:
@PSH@

ANESTHESIA:
Local 1% lidocaine cutaneous anesthetic

Medications:
@MEDENC@
{Blank multiple:19196::"Cefadroxil 500 mg","Cefadroxil 1000 mg","Clindamycin 600 mg","Valium 5 mg", "Valium 10 mg","Lorazepam 0.5 mg","Lorazepam 1 mg":}

Allergies:
@ALG@

VITALS:
@VITALSMULTIPLE@

POST-OP VITALS:
BP:*** Pulse:***

@TIMEOUT@

PROCEDURE START TIME: ***

VCSS: R:*** L:***
CEAP CLASS: Right: {Blank single:19197::"C0","C1","C2","C3","C4","C5","C6"} Left:{Blank single:19197::"C0","C1","C2","C3","C4","C5","C6"}

INDICATIONS:
@DIAG@
Leg pain, swelling, varicose veins, and venous insufficiency in the {Blank single:19197::"right","left","bilateral"} leg {Blank multiple:19196::"great saphenous","anterior great saphenous","small saphenous","posterior thigh extension"} vein system.

FINDINGS:
The treated saphenous vein(s) appeared to be occluded following the cyanoacrylate glue procedure. The common femoral and popliteal veins were normal and compressible after the procedure. There were no phlebitis vein segments.

PROCEDURE:
Duplex ultrasound was used to map out the insufficient saphenous vein, and access was determined and marked on the overlying skin. The depth and diameter of the vein(s) to be treated were documented. The patient was placed supine on the procedure table, and the leg was prepped and draped using sterile technique.

Ultrasound guidance was again used to localize the access site. 1% lidocaine was injected as a local anesthetic in the subcutaneous tissues at the target location in the GSV in the lower leg. Using ultrasound guidance, access was gained at this location with the 19-gauge thin-walled access needle, and followed by introduction of a short guidewire, location confirmed with ultrasound. A small, 3 mm incision was made at the access site to allow for introduction and placement of the 7 Fr ×7cm introducer/dilator. The dilator and guidewire were removed. The 0.035 guidewire from the VenaSeal kit was then introduced and positioned at the saphenofemoral junction using ultrasound guidance. The 80 cm 7 Fr introducer sheath/dilator was positioned 5 cm from the saphenofemoral junction. The guidewire and dilator were removed, and the remaining sheath was flushed with sterile saline, with the syringe remaining in place prior to the next steps.

The cyanoacrylate adhesive was precisely primed into the 5 F delivery catheter, and this catheter/syringe combination was attached within the dispenser gun. This "assembly" was introduced through the 7 Fr sheath and positioned 5 cm caudal to the saphenofemoral junction under ultrasound guidance. *The steps from the IFU were followed for dispensing amounts, locations, and compression times, e.g., 2 aliquots proximally with 3 min of compression, and 1 aliquot every 3 cm distally with 30 s of compression along the course of the vessel.* Following the last injection and compression sequence, the catheter and introducer sheath were pulled out from the access site. Hemostasis was achieved with manual compression, and an adhesive bandage was applied to the incision. Ultrasound confirmed complete coaptation and closure of the treated segments of the GSV, and the absence of any DVT at the saphenofemoral junction.

Vein	Aliquots	Length/CM
***	***	***
***	***	***
***	***	***

The drapes were removed and the patient cleaned and prepared for discharge. Post op ultrasound check is scheduled for 48–72 h and the patient was given written post-op instructions.

PROCEDURE END TIME: ***

DISCHARGE/PLAN:

Estimated blood loss is minimal, all counts were correct, and the patient's prognosis for recovery is good. There were no complications. There were no specimens sent. The patient will leave their compression stocking on until the post-procedure visit and then for the remainder of 2 weeks during waking hours, or as directed by the physician. The patient ambulated upon discharge after having tolerated the procedure well. Oral and written instructions were reviewed with the patient before discharge. The patient was released to *** and will plan to return in 1–2 days for an ultrasound and dressing change. The patient will be scheduled for further injections of PEM (Varithena) as needed for residual varices/truncal reflux in the next 4–6 weeks.

Mechanicochemical Ablation Procedure (MOCA) Note

@NAME@
@MRN@
@ED@

PRE-PROCEDURE DIAGNOSIS: {Blank multiple:19196::"Right","Left","Bilateral"} leg venous insufficiency, leg pain, edema, varicose veins

POST-PROCEDURE DIAGNOSIS: {Blank multiple:19196::"Right","Left","Bilateral"} leg venous insufficiency of the lower extremity

PROCEDURE: {Blank multiple:19196::"Right","Left","Bilateral"} leg transcatheter occlusion of the incompetent {Blank multiple:19196::"Great Saphenous","Anterior Great Saphenous","Small Saphenous","Posterior thigh extension"} vein.

PHYSICIAN: Carlos Echevarria, MD

FELLOW:

ASSISTANT: {Blank multiple:19196::"xyz","abc"}

Surgical History:
@PSH@

ANESTHESIA:
Local 1% lidocaine cutaneous anesthetic

Medications:
@MEDENCOUNTER@
{Blank multiple:19196::"Cefadroxil 500 mg","Cefadroxil 1000 mg","Clindamycin 600 mg","Valium 5 mg", "Valium 10 mg","Lorazepam 0.5 mg","Lorazepam 1 mg":}

Allergies:
@ALG@

VITAL SIGNS:
@VITALSMULTIPLE@

@TIMEOUT@

PROCEDURE START TIME: ***

VCSS: R:*** L:***
CEAP CLASS: Right: {Blank single:19197::"C0","C1","C2","C3","C4","C5","C6"} Left:{Blank single:19197::"C0","C1","C2","C3","C4","C5","C6"}

INDICATIONS: @DIAG@

FINDINGS:
The junction with the deep vein system appeared to be patent.
The treated vein segment appeared to be partially/fully occluded.
There were incompetent perforators adjacent to the vein treated at the *** level.
There were enlarged tributaries coming off of the treated saphenous vein at the ***level.

PROCEDURE: With the patient in the supine/prone position, the patients leg was washed with DuraPrep/ChloraPrep cleanser and draped in the usual sterile manner. The target vein was imaged at the proximal junction where it measured *** mm in diameter. The vein was followed distally with ultrasound to an area at the *** level where it was cannulated percutaneously with a 1% lidocaine skin wheal and a 21-gauge micropuncture needle. Through this needle a series of guidewires and introducers were passed, and ultimately a 5 French micropuncture sheath was placed into the venous system at this level.

Through this catheter, the occlusion catheter was passed up to the saphenous vein junction using ultrasound guidance. The tip was deployed and positioned carefully at 1 cm from the junction. The position was marked with ultrasound guidance.

The occlusion catheter was then turned on, using a rotating wire speed of 3500 revolutions per minute. The catheter was pulled back approximately 1 cm without injection in order to create some venous spasm proximally. Then the catheter was pulled back at approximately 1.5 mm per second with simultaneous slow infusion via the catheter of ***% sodium tetradecyl sulfate liquid solution to attain transcatheter occlusion of the abnormal saphenous vein. At the completion of the pullback, the treated vein was re-imaged with the above findings. Total length of vein treated *** cm. Total solution used ***cc.

PROCEDURE END TIME:***

DISCHARGE: The procedure was considered to be adequate after the interpretation of the ultrasound, and the catheter was then removed and pressure was held for hemostasis at the entry site. The incision was dressed with a Steri-Strip and Tegaderm. A 30 mmHg compression stocking was applied to the thigh high level. The patient was immediately ambulated and was discharged having tolerated the procedure well. Routine follow-up was arranged. There were no complications.

Sclerotherapy (Cosmetic, Medically Necessary, Ultrasound Guided)

Set Up

1 box of 0.5% Asclera (polidocanol)
1 box of 1% Asclera (polidocanol)
1 box of 1% sodium tetradecyl sulfate (STS)
5 syringes
5 18" Needles
5 30 ½″ needles
5 30 1″ needles
5 25″ needles
2 18″ micro filter needles
Alcohol
Cotton balls
Sharps container

Medically Necessary Sclerotherapy Note

@NAME@
@MRN@
@ED@

PROCEDURE DIAGNOSIS:{Blank single:19197::"Right","Left ","Bilateral"} leg venous insufficiency with leg pain, swelling, and varicose veins

PROCEDURE PERFORMED:{Blank single:19197::"Right","Left","Bilateral"} leg medically necessary sclerotherapy

PHYSICIAN: Carlos Echevarria, MD

FELLOW:

ASSISTANT: {Blank single:19197::"xyz ","xyz"}

Surgical History:
@PSH@

Medications:
@MEDENCOUNTER@
{Blank multiple:19196::"Cefadroxil 500 mg","Cefadroxil 1000 mg","Clindamycin 600 mg","Valium 5 mg", "Valium 10 mg","Lorazepam 0.5 mg","Lorazepam 1 mg":}

Allergies:
@ALG@

Vital Signs:
@VS@

Post-Op Vitals:
BP:*** Pulse:***

VCSS: R:*** L:***
CEAP CLASS: Right: {Blank single:19197::"C0","C1","C2","C3","C4","C5","C6"} Left:{Blank single:19197::"C0","C1","C2","C3","C4","C5","C6"}

INDICATIONS:@DIAG@ {Blank single:19197::"Right","Left", "Bilateral"} leg varicose veins of the lower extremity with inflammation

FINDINGS: The symptomatic tributaries in the areas injected.

@TIMEOUT@

PROCEDURE:
The patient was placed in Trendelenburg, in the {Blank multiple:19196:: "supine", "prone", "decubitus"} position. With alcohol preparation and vein light guidance, a 30-gauge needle was used to insert into multiple tributary/reticular veins:

vein treated/area of treatment	cc	form	agent
***	***	{Blank single:19197::"liquid","foam","CO2 foam"}	{Blank single:19197::"0.5% PD","1%PD","1%STS"}
vein treated/area of treatment	cc	form	agent
***	***	{Blank single:19197::"liquid","foam","CO2 foam"}	{Blank single:19197::"0.5% PD","1%PD","1%STS"}

DISCHARGE/PLAN:

Dressings: 30 mmHg compression stockings were immediately put on the patient after injection.

Instructions: Having tolerated the procedure well the patient will continue to wear the compression garment continuously for 48 h and every day following during waking hours for a total of 14 days.

The patient was {Blank single:19197::"ambulated immediately without difficulty" ,"kept in the Trendelenburg position for 30 min following the last foam injection, with calf muscle pumps performed following injections."}

There were no complications.

The patient will plan to return ***. In the meantime, they will call with any questions or if any other issues occur.

Summary

The *non-thermal ablation* workflows outline standardized protocols for minimally invasive venous treatments. These techniques include the use of the following:

Varithena (Polidocanol Microfoam) and details about proper documentation, including treated vein segments, foam volumes, and follow-up instructions.

- *VenaSeal (Cyanoacrylate Glue)*: Adhesive-based closure of refluxing veins via catheter delivery. The setup includes specialized glue kits, ultrasound guidance, and post-op management.
- *MOCA*: Combines mechanical agitation (rotating wire) with a sclerosing agent (STS) to occlude veins. Requires tumescent anesthesia and real-time ultrasound monitoring.
- *Sclerotherapy*: Direct injection of liquid/foam sclerosants (polidocanol, STS) into varicose veins, with compression garment use post-procedure.

All procedures emphasize *sterile technique*, *patient verification*, *ultrasound guidance*, and *post-op compression*. Sedation is optional (with driving restrictions), and follow-up includes duplex ultrasound checks.

Microsurgical Techniques 19

Carlos Echevarria, Sherry D. Scovell,
and Julianne Stoughton

Phlebectomy

Set Up

Veinlite and pen
Small kit
Four drape sheets
Two jakes baby hemostatic forceps
One pair of scissors
One light cover

C. Echevarria
Division of Vascular and Endovascular Surgery, Department of Surgery, Massachusetts General Hospital/Harvard Venous & Lymphatic Medicine Alumni, Boston, MA, USA

Division of Vascular Medicine and Endovenous Interventions, Veins & Vascular Centers of Excellence, Phoenix, AZ, USA
e-mail: carlos.echevarria@vascular.md

S. D. Scovell · J. Stoughton (✉)
Division of Vascular and Endovascular Surgery, Department of Surgery, Massachusetts General Hospital/Harvard Medical School, Boston, MA, USA
e-mail: sscovell@mgh.harvard.edu; jstoughton@mgh.harvard.edu

C. Echevarria et al. (eds.), *The Massachusetts General Hospital Protocols and Procedures for Venous Disease*,
https://doi.org/10.1007/978-3-032-05708-2_19

One package of tubing
One DuraPrep/ChloraPrep
One micro needle
One 25 gauge needle
One pair of sterile gloves
One package of gauze
One ice bag
One elastic
Steri-Strips (as much as needed)
Tegaderm (as much as needed)
One spinal needle (optional)
One fluid bag ready to mix tumescent (includes sodium bicarb and 1% lidocaine with epi)
One gown
One pair of socks
One pair of underwear (men get two pairs)
One large Ace wrap
One goodie bag (small Ace bandage, chux, ABD pad, ice pack, instructions)

Open a small surgical pack first and sterilely place all components on the table at least 5 inches above the sterile field, taking care not to contaminate any of the supplies. It does not matter in which order they are placed on the table. During this procedure, you will need to obtain ice from the machine or freezer (ice in a sterile bag is used for vasoconstriction and pain control). Talk to the patient to keep them calm and relaxed. Make sure there is music the patient prefers or, if not, something soothing (classical is a good go-to).

Make sure the patient is appropriately dressed for the procedure; use the veinlite and marking pen for marking. Ask the patient about meds, allergies, and DOB every time. Sedatives are optional. Patients cannot drive if they have taken sedatives. Identify the designated driver prior to initiating the procedure. Compression hoses are required for every procedure.

Ambulatory Phlebectomy Note

@NAME@
@MRN@
@ED@

PREOPERATIVE DIAGNOSIS: {Blank single:19197::"Right"," Left","Bilateral"} leg venous insufficiency, leg pain, edema, varicose veins

POST-OPERATIVE DIAGNOSIS: Same

PROCEDURE: {Blank single:19197::"Right","Left","Bilateral"} leg ambulatory phlebectomy with *** micro-incisions total

PHYSICIAN: Carlos Echevarria, MD

FELLOW: ***

ASSISTANT: {Blank single:19197::"xyz","xyz"}

Surgical History:
@PSH@

ANESTHESIA: *** mL tumescent local ({Blank multiple:19196::"250 mL 0.09% sodium chloride, 10 cc lidocaine with epinephrine and 2.5 cc sodium bicarbonate","500 mL 0.09% sodium chloride, 20 cc lidocaine with epinephrine and 5 cc sodium bicarbonate"})

Medications:
@MEDENC@
{Blank multiple:19196::"Cefadroxil 500 mg","Cefadroxil 1000 mg","Clindamycin 600 mg","Valium 5 mg","Valium 10 mg","Lorazepam 0.5mg","Lorazepam 1mg":}

Allergies:
@ALG@

VITALS SIGNS:
@VITALSMULTIPLE@

POST-OP VITALS:
BP:*** Pulse:***

@TIMEOUT@

PROCEDURE START TIME:***

VCSS: R:*** L:***
CEAP CLASS: Right:{Blank single:19197::"C0","C1","C2","C3","C4","C5","C6"} Left:{Blank single:19197::"C0","C1","C2","C3","C4","C5","C6"}

INDICATIONS: @DIAG@
leg pain, swelling, varicose veins, and venous insufficiency in the {Blank single:19197::"right","left","bilateral"} lower extremity.
Conservative measures failed (hose, elevation, exercise, medications).

FINDINGS: There were no phlebitic vein segments present.

PROCEDURE:
The patient was placed in Trendelenburg in the {Blank single:19197::"supine","prone","left lateral decubitus","right lateral decubitus"} position on the operating table. The {Blank single:19197::"right","left","bilateral"} leg was prepped with {Blank single:19197::"duraprep","chloraprep"} and draped sterilely. The previously marked varicose veins of the {Blank single:19197::"right","left","bilateral"} leg were infused with tumes-

cent anesthesia, a total of *** micro-incisions were made to remove the symptomatic varicosities in the following areas;***.

All the incisions were dressed with Steri-Strips and Tegaderm. ABD pads were placed over each incision site and a 30 mmHg compression stocking ({Blanksingle:19197::"Thigh high with waist attachment","thigh high","pantyhose","knee high"}) was applied on the patient. An additional Ace bandage was applied over the stockings up to the high-thigh level, to be taken off prior to bed time.

PROCEDURE END TIME:***

DISCHARGE:

Estimated blood loss was minimal. All counts were correct, and the patient's prognosis for recovery is good. There were no complications, and no specimens were sent.

The patient will leave their compression stocking on until the post-procedure visit and then for an additional 2 weeks during waking hours, or as directed by the physician. The patient ambulated upon discharge after having tolerated the procedure well. Oral and written instructions were reviewed with the patient prior to discharge. The patient was released to *** and will is scheduled to return in 1–2 days for an ultrasound and dressing change.

Microthrombectomy

Set Up

Ultrasound (if needed)
Veinlite
Lidocaine 1%
3 cc syringes with needle
Two micro filter needles, 18″
Alcohol

Cotton balls
2 × 2 gauze
Bacitracin
Tape
Sharps container

Microthrombectomy Note

?
@NAME@
@MRN@
@ED@

PROCEDURE DIAGNOSIS:
{Blank single:19197::"Right","Left","Bilateral"} leg intraluminal thrombus, leg pain post-treatment
?
POST-PROCEDURE DIAGNOSIS:
Same
?
PROCEDURE PERFORMED:
{Blank single:19197::"Right","Left","Bilateral"} leg micro-thrombectomy
{Blank single:19197::"Varithena Foam","Cosmetic sclerotherapy","Medically Necessary Sclerotherapy"} performed on ***
?
PHYSICIAN: Carlos Echevarria, MD

FELLOW:

ASSISTANT: {Blank single:19197::"xyz","abc"}?
?
Surgical History:

@PSH@

?

ANESTHESIA: {Blank single:19197::"Local","None"}

Medications:

??@MEDENCOUNTER@

?

Allergies:

@ALG@

?

VITAL SIGNS:

?@VITALSMULTIPLE@

??

INDICATIONS: Intraluminal thrombus with pain and swelling

?@DIAG@

FINDINGS: There is intraluminal thrombus in the ***

@TIMEOUT@

PROCEDURE:

Palpable collections were identified subcutaneously on the {Blank single:19197::"right","left","bilateral"} leg. The patient was placed in the {Blank multiple:19196::"supine","prone","decub itus"} position. After alcohol preparation, a 1% lidocaine wheal was performed and an 18-gauge needle was used to puncture multiple veins in the {Blank single:19197::"right","l eft","bilateral"} {Blank multiple:19196::"medial","lateral","a nterior","posterior"} {Blank multiple:19196::"thigh","calf","a nkle"}. The thrombus was {Blank single:19197::"partially","f ully"} evacuated in these areas without difficulty. A 2 × 2 gauze with bacitracin was placed over each site and secured with paper tape.

DISCHARGE/PLAN:

The patient was counseled on wound care and discharged ambulatory. The patient will follow up with the physician for further procedures as scheduled, or sooner if the hematoma returns.

Summary

The *microsurgical* workflows detail minimally invasive procedures for treating varicose veins and post-treatment thrombi. This chapter details proper setup and reporting of the following:

- *Phlebectomy*: Small incisions are made to remove superficial varicose veins under tumescent anesthesia. Setup includes a sterile kit (Veinlite, micro-needles, dressings), patient verification, and post-op compression therapy (30 mmHg stockings). Documentation covers incision sites, anesthesia volume, and follow-up care.
- *Microthrombectomy*: Evacuates painful intraluminal thrombi (e.g., post-sclerotherapy) via needle aspiration. Requires lidocaine, ultrasound (if needed), and sterile gauze dressings.

Both procedures emphasize *sterile technique*, *patient comfort*, and *compression therapy*. Discharge instructions include activity guidelines and follow-up ultrasounds.

Index

C. Echevarria et al. (eds.), *The Massachusetts General Hospital Protocols and Procedures for Venous Disease*, https://doi.org/10.1007/978-3-032-05708-2

MIX
Papier aus verantwortungsvollen Quellen
Paper from responsible sources
FSC® C105338

If you have any concerns about our products,
you can contact us on
ProductSafety@springernature.com

In case Publisher is established outside the EU,
the EU authorized representative is:
Springer Nature Customer Service Center GmbH
Europaplatz 3, 69115 Heidelberg, Germany

Printed by Libri Plureos GmbH
in Hamburg, Germany